SIGNS OF LIFE II

D1572442

SIGNS OF LIFE II

By Mark Mosier,
Mobile Intensive Care Paramedic

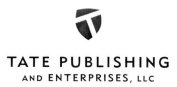

TATE PUBLISHING
AND ENTERPRISES, LLC

Published by Tate Publishing & Enterprises, LLC
127 E. Trade Center Terrace | Mustang, Oklahoma 73064 USA
1.888.361.9473 | www.tatepublishing.com

Tate Publishing is committed to excellence in the publishing industry. The company reflects the philosophy established by the founders, based on Psalm 68:11,
"The Lord gave the word and great was the company of those who published it."

Book design copyright © 2016 by Tate Publishing, LLC. All rights reserved.
Cover design by Samson Lim
Interior design by Mary Jean Archival

Published in the United States of America

ISBN: 978-1-68254-883-7
Medical / Emergency Medicine
16.01.28

CONTENTS

PREFACE

STATION 4 IS one of the busiest EMS (Emergency Medical Services) departments in the county. When a person calls 9-1-1, something significant has taken place, and odds are probably not in the patient's favor. There will be chaos, panic, and more often than not, the crew starting behind the proverbial eight ball.

Maybe it's a car crash where someone is pinned, a heart attack victim who stops breathing, a patient with a massive stroke, or heroin addict who stops breathing after an overdose. Whatever the crew is faced with, they'll bring the highest competence, professionalism, and compassion along with the skills and equipment to make *some* difference on every call. It's an impressive response.

In EMS, we rely on the public. They are the first links in the chain of survival, recognizing an emergency exists, early access to 9-1-1 and providing any care they're capable of or willing which can have profound influences in outcomes. Minutes can literally shift the balance between life and death.

Last month, a man suffered a heart attack while driving in the middle of downtown. He lost consciousness as his car came to rest against a curb. A few feet away, a couple we're sitting on a park bench, relaxing and enjoying the day. Unexpectedly, they became the central element in this life-and-death encounter playing out right in front of them.

They could see the man was having a medical issue as he was slumped over the steering wheel and not moving. One of them placed an immediate call to 9-1-1 while the other was able to get him out the car onto the sidewalk.

The patient's face rapidly turned blue; he was taking short gasping-type breaths, and suddenly in cardiac arrest. The bystander began CPR. This was continued for four minutes until the ambulance and rescue squad arrived and took over care.

After two shocks with the defibrillator, his pulse was restored and transported to the hospital. He underwent heart bypass surgery and discharged home ten days later.

Does this mean everyone who gets help from a citizen will have that *miracle outcome*? No, but it certainly improves their chances. Had the couple chosen *not* to get involved, the result would almost certainly have been different.

This was an incredible success story. The couple never considered themselves anything more than, "Happy to be in the right place at the right time."

My paramedic mentor here at Station 4 gave me a quote many years ago which I still reflect on today: "Every call is a chance to make a difference in someone's life."

The *Signs of Life II* stories are based on actual responses. Welcome to Station 4. Let's go see what kind of differences we can make.

DISCLAIMER

HAVE A SEAT, buckle up, and find something to hang on to. You're in for quite a ride. I want to give you the same *heads-up* I give all riders. We may see and do some things that can be pretty intense. You'll look at life a little differently after this day. It's okay to take a break and walk away for a few minutes. And one more thing, you wouldn't be human if some of these stories…well, you'll see!

1

OUR EXTENDED FAMILY

STATION 4 IS located in the heart of the city. On an average day, it isn't uncommon for the crews to respond to fifteen calls in a twenty-four hour period. The response area covers short response times in the urban city to extended response in the rural expanses. Station 4 is a *combo department*, which means we're staffed by both career personnel and dedicated first responder and EMT volunteers.

Sandy Martin is the Station 4 administrative secretary. She's been with the department for fifteen years. Sandy is as proficient in her position as the crews are at dealing with the daily life and death challenges they can face. She's the reason things run as efficiently as they do and is unchallenged in that role. From dealing with the public or station personnel, it all goes through and is resolved by Sandy.

"Paramedic Mark Mosier, could you please come to my office," Sandy called out over the intercom.

We had just come on duty for the day. The truck bay is alive with activity inspecting the rigs and checking equipment.

"Nice knowing you," Rocky called out while poking his head from inside the ambulance and flashing a better-thee-than-me, grin.

"I thought partners watched each other's back," I said with an imploring expression.

"Moral support, man, I got you covered," he replied.

I started that lonely walk through the truck bay into the front offices.

"Hi, Sandy, what's up?" I asked.

"Do you remember Mr. Freeman from last week?" she asked.

"Sure, that was the toughest call of the shift, it didn't matter what we did he wasn't happy," I explained.

That fateful day, Mr. Freeman called 9-1-1 complaining of general aches and pains, sick, possibly ill, and requesting transport to the hospital. When we arrived, he was sitting in his wheelchair at the end of his driveway with two suitcases next to him, staring at his watch and shaking his head.

"Took you seven minutes to get here," he complained. "What if I was dying?" he added angrily.

That was the easiest part of the call as it went downhill from there.

Sandy looked at me with an empathetic grin and said, "Well, Mr. Freeman's being discharged from the hospital today and wants to know where his wheelchair and keys to his house are."

This caused an involuntary sigh, nodding of the head, and right hand to the forehead partially covering my right eye.

"His neighbor has both the wheelchair and the keys, which were his *very* specific instructions," I explained defensively.

Back to the truck bay where I thanked Rocky for the *moral support* to which he replied, "No problem, man, that's what partners are for."

Rocky and I have been partners since I became a paramedic eight years ago. The time has gone fast. I vividly remember walking through that front door, meeting Sandy, and beginning a journey and career that would be difficult to script.

Jim "Rocky" Rocha is a veteran EMT and excellent partner. His wife Rachel is a nurse in the emergency department at Regional General Hospital.

Regional, or RGH as we call it, is a level-one trauma center. There's no higher level of care beyond what Regional provides. This is our primary destination for transports.

Rocky and Rachel have three dogs that might as well be their kids—Hank, a black lab; Abby, a black and white springer spaniel/lab mix; and Kelsey, a golden retriever. Rachel brings them to visit the station often and it's never a dull moment. I'm sure the dogs wonder why we don't all live together.

"Where's the rescue crew this morning?" I asked Rocky.

"They're finishing the early morning class for the volunteers," he said as if I should have known that.

There are three main parts to EMS: running calls, paperwork, and training; and not always in that order.

Steve Risley and Dana Davidson walked out the training room followed by several first responder volunteers. Steve presented a training class on long spine board application and extremity splinting. Dana was the "patient" for the training and looked like she had all the fun she wanted for one day. She was splinted and packaged, and splinted and packaged.

Dana was recently hired on full time as a career EMT. She had been an active volunteer for ten years prior and works part time as a pediatric nurse at Regional. As a career EMT, Dana works a twenty-four-hour shift followed by two days off. Dana fills a role on Rescue 41 that was vacated by Eric Wright. Eric worked with us for several years before taking the step to paramedic and then transferred to a neighboring station.

We tell Eric we miss him dearly but in fact I think we'll keep Dana.

Dana is barely over five feet tall. Don't let Dana's size mislead you, she's one of the strongest EMTs we have on our crew, literally and figuratively. Her smile is infectious and she shares it generously.

Steve Risley is a career EMT and captain on Rescue 41. He's been with Station 4 for just over fifteen years. With prior military experience, there isn't much Steve isn't capable of. Steve is our "go to guy" for some of the best cooking which we take full advantage of and are treated to often.

Samantha "Sam" Grieves is the third member of Rescue 41. She is also a well-seasoned career EMT and an integral part of our success. She's been with Station 4 nearly ten years. At just a couple inches taller than Dana, they share uncanny similarities that could make them sisters; in the EMS world, they are.

Last month, Sam was recognized by the State EMS council and awarded EMT of the Year. This got her a plaque proudly displayed in our dayroom and complimenting article in the newspaper along with having to buy ice cream for the station. Anytime you get ink, you have to buy ice cream. We don't invent the traditions, we just follow them.

Rescue 41 is a crew cab heavy-duty pickup truck that's dispatched along with Rocky and I in the ambulance, Medic 42. With the three-person crew of Steve, Sam, and Dana, the manpower they bring to the scene is vital to our success. They carry additional equipment used for those multiple-patient scenarios. On most calls, Sam and Dana will accompany the transport to the hospital with Rocky and I, while Steve will follow with the Rescue to bring them back to the station.

And I'm Mark Mosier, the career paramedic in charge for this group. I've been a paramedic for the last eight years and here at Station 4 for the past ten years. All our crew members are among the best of the best at their roles. We're not successful because of one person: we're successful because we're a strong and committed team.

Not to be excluded, we couldn't provide the same level of service without our dedicated volunteers of first responder and EMTs. We have a proactive group willing to ensure coverage is complete. Occasionally, some of them will join Rocky and I on Medic 42, as a third person. Not only does this provide additional help with patient care but also it's hands-on experience they can't get from classroom training.

Our volunteers have full-time jobs outside the department in the community, it's not uncommon to arrive on a scene and find one them providing initial and ongoing care.

Last month, Rocky and I responded to a patient who had passed out at the dentist's office. We arrived to find Ariel, one of our volunteers, kneeling at the top of the patient's head with her hands alongside his ears. She is holding in-line immobilization due to a potential cervical spine (neck) injury and greeted us with a confident smile.

Ariel works as a dental hygienist in the office and witnessed the patient collapsed and fall quite violently head first into a wall. This was great information and initial patient care. She also had to "interpret" for the patient who received local anesthesia. We had trouble understanding the "slurred" verbal responses.

Another one of our volunteers became a star when she faced a life-and-death emergency which unfolded literally right in front of her.

The ever familiar Station 4 tones from our 9-1-1 center resonated throughout the station coming from the overhead ceiling speakers sending us to her with the precarious dispatch.

"Rescue 41, Medic 42, respond code three for cardiac arrest, CPR in progress, 1801 Hanford Street, Express Cleaners time out 1016 hours."

This will be a four-minute response with traffic. It isn't far from here, but we have the challenge of city driving and traffic lights along with the ubiquitous distracted drivers. Code three driving, which is lights and siren, is extremely hazardous and more so in congestion. If we crash before we arrive, we don't make the situation any better!

Rocky is navigating through the gauntlet of traffic with ease.

Pulling up in front of the business, we're met by an employee nervously standing on the sidewalk waving several times to ensure we see him.

"Please hurry, I think he had a heart attack," he said with serious certainty and near panic.

"Okay, lead the way," I said.

Rescue 41 arrived with us, and after quickly grabbing all our equipment, we head into the front door of the business.

We have several pieces of essential equipment to bring with us. We have the LifePak 12 or cardiac monitor, the main kit with emergency medications and IV supplies, an airway kit for any breathing issues, portable suction for vomiting, and a portable oxygen bottle.

We're literally bringing the emergency department to your front door.

There's a male in his fifties on the floor next to the front counter.

CPR is being performed by a female, and as I walked over, she looked up and said, "Hi, Mark, I was here picking up clothes, this guy grabbed his chest and hit the ground. I started CPR right away."

It's Katrina, one of our stronger EMT volunteers and most active CPR instructor. She's sweating profusely; her hair is matted against her face after doing continual chest compressions for the last five minutes.

There are streaks and chunks of vomit in her hair from when the patient vomited during one of the breaths she administered between compressions. There's another large pile several feet away and quite aromatic. She effectively rolled the patient onto his side during the vomiting episode preventing him from aspirating, and then pulled him clear of the pile in order to continue CPR.

Aspiration is any liquid or solids going into the lungs. When a person is unconscious or in cardiac arrest, they're at risk for this as they cannot protect their airway.

"Steve, take over for Katrina on compressions, Sam, you and Dana got the airway," I said.

Steve nodded and was quickly at the patient's side displaying textbook form as he's done hundreds of times before.

Sam grabbed the bag valve mask out of the airway kit. She placed the mask portion over the patient's mouth and nose and held it firmly. Dana squeezed the bag and the man's chest rose as air filled his lungs.

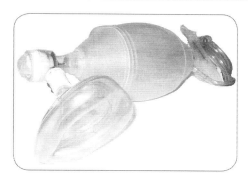

This is the bag valve mask or BVM. It's used to provide breaths for a patient not breathing. The mask portion is fitted over the mouth and nose and bag is squeezed to introduce air into the lungs. It can be used by one or two people, it's easier with two. Once the patient is intubated (breathing tube placed), the mask piece is removed and the bag valve attaches to the adapter on the end of the breathing tube.

Katrina moved backward into a sitting position on the floor against the wall with her hands on her knees and let out a deep sigh.

"Thanks for the quick response, you guys. I was just about done," she said, her lip quivering with emotion.

"Hey, no problem, Katrina, you did perfect!" I said encouragingly.

Rocky applied the large rectangular adhesive "fast patches" on the patient's chest and plugged the wires into the LifePak 12 which would allow us to see the (electrocardiogram) EKG rhythm the patient is in.

He's working around Steve who is focused on delivering compressions. We have several things going on at the exact same time and working as if it were a choreographed performance rehearsed over and over and over.

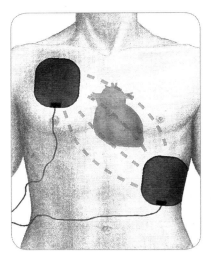

The fast patches are applied to the chest during cardiac arrest. These patches plug into the LifePak 12 and allow us to see the cardiac rhythm or EKG. The shock or defibrillation is delivered through them. One is placed in the right upper chest and the other to the left lower chest region.

"Stop compressions, Steve," I ordered as we all focused on the screen of the LifePak 12.

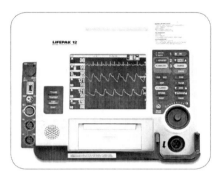

The LifePak 12 is our cardiac monitor. We use it for any cardiac or heart-related emergency. It's capable of displaying the EKG activity or rhythm of the heart and can deliver a life-saving defibrillation through the fast patches if needed during cardiac arrest. We can also get a 12-lead EKG which can show us a heart attack in progress or measure automatic blood pressures and much more. (Photo courtesy of Physio Control)

"V-fib, we'll charge to 200 and shock, clear," and the shock was delivered with the patient arching to the energy of it.

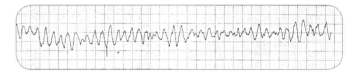

This is ventricular fibrillation, or V-fib. The heart is quivering, no pulse is being generated. We have to deliver a shock from the LifePak 12 with the goal of stopping all this activity. This will potentially allow the heart to start beating in a normal rhythm. We'll deliver one shock every two minutes with increasing energy levels as long as V-fib persists with CPR performed in between.

The delivered energy is measured in watt seconds, or joules. It's definitely enough to cause a notable *jump* by anyone who receives the shock. We generally just call out the number, "200 or 300 or 360" and leave the joules or watt seconds part off.

"Dana, take over on CPR," I said.

"Roger that," Dana said, and with her small stature, began delivering perfect form compressions with her short brown hair bouncing in synch.

Rocky has the main kit open and getting IV equipment and medications ready as I'm searching for a vein. I find a suitable one on the right mid arm and ensured the IV was securely taped in place. More than one IV has been inadvertently pulled out on a scene with all the activity going on. This will generally happen only once, maybe twice in your career. After that, you'll make sure to use plenty of tape and watch the IV carefully.

The store owner came to me with information about the patient.

"His name is Mr. Seavers. He's a regular customer. He told me he didn't feel well and was going home to rest. He was pale and sweaty and just grabbed his chest and collapsed to the floor. She started CPR.

"Is he going to be okay?" he asked with empathy and disbelief.

"Well, we're working on getting his heart started. If he is, it'll be thanks to Katrina," I added.

It was time to check the rhythm again.

"Okay, stop CPR, Dana, Steve, switch with Dana after this shock," I called out.

"Roger that," Steve and Dana replied nearly in unison while nodding affirmatively.

"Still V-fib, let's shock at 300," I said.

"Clear," I announced as the shock is delivered followed by the familiar muscular body contraction.

"Dana, push the epinephrine, I'm going to get him intubated," I said and moved to the top of the patient's head.

We use (intravenous) IV epinephrine to try to stimulate cardiac activity, make the heart respond to the shocks. Between the CPR, defibrillation, and medication, we hope this will give us ROSC or return of spontaneous circulation, a pulse.

The intubation involves putting an endotracheal tube, or breathing tube down the throat and into the trachea. It requires a laryngoscope which has a long stainless steel blade with a light on the tip which goes into the back of the throat in search of the epiglottis.

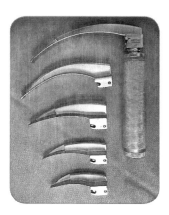

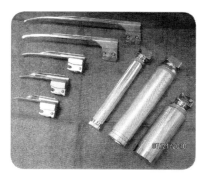

The laryngoscope handles different-size stainless steel blades. My preference is the large curved one. Users should be proficient using both. There's no real advantage; it's based on the medic's preference.

Right below the epiglottis is the vocal cords and opening to the trachea. The endotracheal tube will go between the vocal cords and into the trachea a couple inches. The bag valve would then be attached to the end of the tube and the ventilations or breaths will go directly into the lungs.

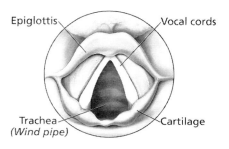

National Cancer Institute

This is the view I have as I look down the patient's throat from above their head. The epiglottis is a "flapper" that protects the trachea from aspiration during swallowing. I will use the laryngoscope blade to "lift" the epiglottis and expose the vocal cords and opening to the trachea.

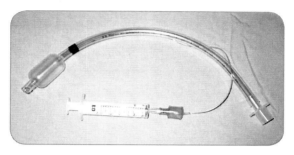

This is the endotracheal tube. It protects the lungs from aspiration (liquid or solids going into the lungs). The end with the "balloon" goes into the trachea and seals it off. The syringe is used to inflate the "balloon" with air after the tube is inserted through the tracheal opening. The mask from the bag valve is removed and the tube attaches to it, when the bag is squeezed, air is introduced directly into the lungs.

The intubation went smoothly and just after I secured the endotracheal tube, Katrina spoke up.

"Mark, his arm's moving," she exclaimed.

That's when we all noticed him moving, we have a pulse back!

"Let's check the rhythm," I called out.

"Very nice, we have a good-looking EKG rhythm and strong carotid pulse," I said.

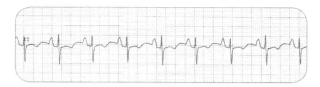

This is what we always hope to see, a regular rhythm.
Notice the difference between this and the V-fib? On this
rhythm, each of the downward spikes is a heartbeat.

"Heart rate 85, blood pressure 96/54, and SpO2 95%," Dana called out.

The SpO2 is a measurement of the amount of oxygen being carried in the red blood cells to the tissues. This is a critical vital sign we monitor closely.

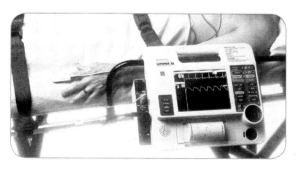

To measure SpO2, the "thimble" looking device goes on a
finger. It then plugs into the LifePak 12 and gives the reading
on the screen. We want the SpO2 to be over 94%. If it drops
below this, we administer supplemental oxygen in order to
increase the percentage. (Photo courtesy of Physio Control)

"Great job, everyone. Let's get him secured to the gurney and head to RGH," I said.

I turned to Katrina and thanked her again for her efforts in this resuscitation.

"Can I come to the hospital with you guys," she asked.

"Sure, you're more than welcome," I said and held out a hand to assist her up.

Mr. Seavers continued to stabilize during the transport. His blood pressure came up and started trying to take some breaths on his own. These are positive signs. We transferred care to the awaiting cardiac team at Regional. He was taken to the coronary cath lab and had two stents put in and admitted to the CCU or coronary care unit.

Stents are a little wire mesh device inserted into a blocked coronary artery in the heart which keep them open and restores circulation and can minimize heart muscle damage.

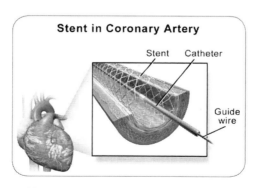

Photo courtesy of BruceBlaus Blausen.com

Mr. Seavers was discharged from the hospital after eight days and returned home to his wife and twin eleven-year-old girls. He was fortunate to not suffer permanent damage. Mr. Seavers got an incredible gift that day, Katrina!

Katrina was recognized by the EMS council and presented with a Citizens Lifesaving Award. Katrina is representative of the caliber of volunteers throughout the EMS system.

Now during her CPR classes, when students ask if CPR actually works, she smiles and says, "Let me tell you a quick story."

The county sponsors an annual rodeo and draws large crowds from out of town. Today's the big day for finals in barrel racing. We might see a few extra calls from the venue, overexertion, trips and falls, but generally a safe and fun time for everyone.

Rocky and I came on duty and barely got the morning rig checks started before the tones started our day.

"Rescue 41, Medic 42, respond code three for a thirty-six-year-old female with difficulty breathing, 1200 Old Farmington Road at the horse arena, time out 0822 hours."

The fairgrounds are about six minutes from the station. Traffic is moderate and it will take every bit of the six-minute response.

"Rescue 41, Medic 42, be advised this is being described as a traumatic injury, there are EMS personnel on scene with the patient at this time."

Steve and I both acknowledged the updated information. We're only a couple minutes away and of course traffic is heavier as we get closer to the arena.

We arrive at the front gate and met by a lone security guard; he's directing us to the arena.

We walked into the large hangar-type building and quickly met by Shannon who, with her husband Roland, are both Station 4 volunteer emergency medical technicians or EMTs.

"Hi, Mark, nice to see you guys," Shannon said with relief and hint of urgency.

"Roland is with the patient. Her horse rolled on top of her, and we think she may have some broken ribs, she's hurting really bad," she explained as we walked toward the stall.

"Well thanks for being here, Shannon," I said.

Around the corner and into a large stall, we find the patient lying on the ground presenting in obvious extreme distress, struggling with each breath.

Roland is kneeling next to her counting her pulse at the wrist. He has a stethoscope around his neck and small kit with equipment next to him.

Some of the volunteers carry basic first aid kits with a bag valve mask/BVM, blood pressure cuff, and assorted trauma supplies.

"Hi, Mark, she's getting more and more short of breath. I can't hear breath sounds on the left side," Roland said.

"Thanks, Roland, if you want to stay and help we'd appreciate it," I said.

Continuing the initial visual assessment, she's having severe breathing difficulties and laboring to get air in. She has circumoral cyanosis, which is blueness around her lips, blood around her left nare or nostril, and left eye is nearly swollen shut. Additionally, she looks terrified with the respiratory distress she's experiencing.

We would learn the patient's name is Reba. She's thirty-six years old and was scheduled to be part of the competition later today. She finished practicing her routine and was knocked down as her horse tripped. It then fell directly onto her chest and head. She was unconscious for several minutes afterward.

Sam is at Reba's head and has an oxygen mask over her mouth and nose. Dana is holding Reba's head gently in line for spinal precautions. Steve is cutting her shirt off and there's significant bruising over the entire upper left chest. There's obvious deformity along several of the ribs.

Rocky has our kit open and getting equipment ready.

I can't hear breath sounds with my stethoscope in the left chest as she tries to get a breath. I believe she has a pneumothorax that's becoming a tension pneumothorax. This means her collapsed lung is building pressure in the chest, and she'll die from it unless we correct it quickly. This will involve putting a large needle into her chest to relieve this pressure.

I can feel rice krispies under the skin on the left side of the chest. This is air that has leaked into the surrounding tissues creating a *crackling* sensation when you press over it.

The actual medical term for this is subcutaneous emphysema; rice krispies is the slang term and easier to say.

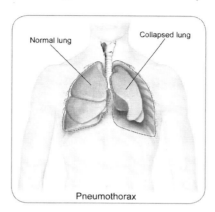

"Her heart rate is 130 and blood pressure is 76/46," Roland said.

This heart rate and accompanying blood pressure indicates Reba is going downhill fast. Without immediate intervention, she may not survive.

Any heart rate over 100 is suspicious, especially with a traumatic injury; it's one of the first vital signs to reflect bleeding internally. For comparison purposes, *normal* heart rates are from 60–90 beats a minute. And a *normal* blood pressure would be like 120/80.

I looked at Reba and said, "Reba, I know you can hear me, don't try to talk, I'm going to put a needle into your chest and this will help you breathe easier."

Reba stared at me, unable to respond. She blinked once; her fear level is at the extreme.

Rocky handed me the big needle which is a 12 gauge, 3-inch long needle. We have designated this as the big needle because it *is* a big needle and used for just this scenario.

I have the insertion landmarks plotted out, midline with the clavicle (collarbone) and between the second and third ribs.

Reba winces and instinctively shrugs her left arm as the needle goes through her chest and hisses loudly for several seconds before going silent. Reba is no longer struggling for breaths but grimacing in pain from the fractured ribs.

We just bought her some time.

Rocky has the LifePak 12 hooked up and calling out the first readings.

"Heart rate 132, blood pressure 74/44, SpO2 at 90%," he said.

We're still seeing the high heart rate and accompanying low blood pressure, and low SpO2. The SpO2 should be over 94%. Reba is in classic blood loss shock.

"Roger that, we can get her secured to the long spine board now," I said.

Reba is looking more alert and trying to talk, but her efforts are only partial whispers. Sam finally realizes she's asking about her horse, Fallon.

"He's fine," Roland said and then tipped his head and winked.

This brought a partial smile and look of relief from Reba.

As Roland and the crew got Reba secured to the spine board and headed to the ambulance, I had a moment to meet with Shannon.

"Thanks for you and Roland being here and helping," I told her with sincerity.

"We're here with friends and were in the next stall and heard the commotion," Shannon explained.

"Station 4 saves the day again," I said with a prideful smile and headed for the ambulance.

I need to get a couple IVs in Reba. I'm worried she may have ruptured her spleen and bleeding from vessels in the chest. She's still critical, as we believe; we only bought her some time.

I placed rubber tourniquets to both her arms, above the elbows.

I will use the first vein that pops up and try to get the biggest IV catheter in the vein will support. The 14 gauge is the largest peripheral IV we can put in a vein. Peripheral veins are the ones in the hands and arms and the jugular vein on the side of the neck is also in this group. The saying for IVs in the prehospital arena is, "Go big or go home".

Reba has two large veins that become immediately visible, one on the right midarm and one on the left midarm. They both get 14 gauges in them. I couldn't help but notice Reba shoot me an evil look after each one was inserted.

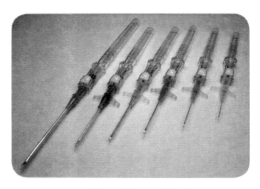

These are our catheters. From left to right, they are 14 gauge, 16 gauge, 18 gauge, 20 gauge, 22 gauge, and the small one is the 24 gauge. Whether they are big or small, all IVs can be painful.

We'll infuse the IV fluids (normal saline) with a goal of getting her blood pressure to at least the eighty range. We don't want to *normalize* her pressure as this could precipitate more bleeding. New standards in prehospital care for internal bleeding include being very cautious and judicious with infusing fluid.

"Heart rate at 120, blood pressure is 82/54, SpO2 92%," Dana called out.

"Okay, sounds good, let's slow the lines down, Sam," I said.

Sam nodded and adjusted the rollers on the IV tubing. We're less than one minute from RGH, just where Reba needs to be.

We arrived at RGH and are directed to suite 12 in the emergency department or ED. Suite 12 is the main trauma room and where the trauma team was standing by.

The trauma team consists of highly skilled nurses, the emergency physician, a trauma surgeon, respiratory therapy, ED techs, lab personnel, all working to get the patient to the next level of care, maybe the (operating room) OR, and then to the ICU or intensive care unit. It's a very impressive performance with the best of the best; the patient cannot get a higher level of care than a level-one trauma center.

Reba had a chest tube placed into her left lateral chest within minutes of our arrival. A chest tube is nearly the size of a small garden hose and inserted into the side of the chest. This will be instrumental in reinflating the lung and removing any blood that may have accumulated secondary to the injury. The insertion area is numbed and then scalpel is used to create the opening for the chest tube.

Her x-rays are impressive with a fractured (broken) sternum and four fractured ribs. She's off to the OR for her spleen laceration.

After ninety minutes, Reba is admitted to the trauma ICU on a ventilator for the next twenty-four hours. She also has a fractured left orbit just below the eye. No barrel racing for a few months but the prognosis for full recovery is excellent.

Once again our volunteers shined and made a difference.

2

NO SLOW DAYS

Rocky and I came on duty at 0800 and by 1000 had four transports. It's not like one of the days of the week is busier than any other. Any day has the potential to be out of control and today just happened to start off that way.

We got back to the station just in time for the day's training. With the dynamics involved with prehospital care, ongoing training is essential to staying sharp each and every time we respond. We divide the time between classroom and practical sessions.

Joey "Joe" Capthorn is the Station 4 EMS and training captain. He's a paramedic and one of, if not, *the* best in the county. He's been a paramedic for the past seventeen years and my mentor when I walked through that front door ten years ago. Much, if not all, of my style comes from Joe. I would call him a paramedic's paramedic.

Brandon Dawson is an EMT and Joe's partner. They've been working together for almost ten years. Brandon was hired on full time a few years ago after working as a shift volunteer. Brandon recently joined the (Special Weapons and Tactics Team) SWAT team as the medic and member on their entry teams. The SWAT guys call him one of "THEM," a tactical hazardous entry medic. He fits this new endeavor in on his days off, and they're fortunate to have Brandon as he is an excellent EMT.

With Sam being our resident firearms expert and competitive shooter, she's been giving Brandon lessons at the range and it has turned into a friendly competition. Brandon has a long ways to go as Sam is nationally ranked at her level.

Brandon is infamous with his near-perfect hair and trademark smile. It doesn't matter how bad your day might be going, spend five minutes with Brandon and you'll quickly find yourself looking at things with a renewed perspective.

He also gets more phone calls than any four of us here at the station. Sandy has threatened more than once to start billing him for the personal secretary role she ends up in. All the calls are from young females; of course Brandon always describes it as "business related."

Joe and Brandon staff Medic 41 and run second out calls. Today, our training would be put on hold after a chilling dispatch has the crews headed for the truck bays.

"Rescue 41, Medic 42, respond code three for a plane crash, in the field behind 8320 Laurel Springs Road, time out 1016."

This wasn't a dispatch we heard too often, and I've only been to one other plane crash, a small single-engine craft that resulted with a double fatality.

Rescue 41 was first out, Dana is driving, and Sam is seated behind Steve in the heavy-duty crew cab Rescue unit. Steve was quickly on the radio inquiring about further information in case we'd need additional resources.

Dispatch immediately provided an important update.

"Medic 42, Rescue 41, this is being described as an ultralight craft. You have one patient who is unconscious at this time, police on scene requesting code three response."

Both Steve and I acknowledged the information. It will take four minutes to arrive. There are two police cars responding in front of us which created the illusion like we're chasing the cops.

We arrived and a police officer is directing us to a dirt road leading to the back of a large barn.

The ultralight craft is demolished and *looked* like a plane crash. It's upside down with twisted pieces of the wings and cockpit strewn about along with smoldering parts of the engine block.

The patient is laying face up about twenty feet away from the center of the crash. From the initial presentation, we see he has obvious fractures to both femurs at midthigh. The left leg is the worst with his left foot being near his head. The right femur is grotesquely folded backward.

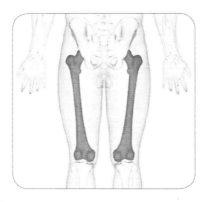

The femur bones are the largest "long" bones in the body. Great force is required to fracture one of these. When both of them are fractured, or broken, we know significant forces were involved and suspect severe injuries associated with this presentation.

A bystander is kneeling at the patient's head holding cervical immobilization and moving side to side as if he is avoiding the front of the patient's face.

I make eye contact with him as I walk up and he says, "I saw him crash, got here right after it happened, he hasn't moved and keeps moaning, I just held his head straight, and he's really gagging from that jaw."

"Okay, thanks for helping, Sam, you and Dana take over for him and see if you can keep that airway open for a few minutes," I directed.

The patient must have gone face first into something on the panel of the ultralight.

His jaw is grossly deformed and fractured with the left side awkwardly hanging down by a couple inches. It's elongating the mouth. There's a full-thickness laceration going from the left corner of the mouth, down along the neck to the left collarbone, it's gaping and I fortunately don't see any spurting blood.

The tongue is severed and part of it's dangling along the jaw. Blood is draining into the back of the throat creating spray as he coughs every few seconds.

Sam realigned the jaw as Dana is using the portable suction perfectly as evidenced by the gagging has stopped.

Rocky has a large trauma dressing secured to the gaping neck wound and taped in place.

"Steve, I need you to get the clothes cut and those femurs stabilized, let's get the (medical antishock trousers) MAST pants on," I said.

"Roger that," Steve replied and withdrew his trauma scissors from his belt holster, twirled them once and began cutting.

MAST pants are a specialized set of *trousers* that go over the legs and up to the lower abdomen. They're a heavy-duty nylon suit with sewn-in air bags in each leg and abdominal section. These can be inflated with air and act as splints and perfect for these types of injuries. Each section can be inflated individually as needed.

This patient is classified as a "multisystem trauma." This means his injuries involve multiple areas of the body and are life-threatening. His condition warrants aggressive yet competent treatment and expeditious transport to a higher level of care which is RGH.

Fortunately, the crew has brought those skills today.

I started at the head and began my assessment to map out a treatment plan. Securing the airway will be priority one.

In addition to the oral injuries and bleeding from the mouth, he's bleeding out both ears and has periorbital ecchymosis or deep bluish discoloration under both eyes. We call this raccoon eyes because it resembles a raccoon face.

The bleeding out the ears and periorbital ecchymosis can be associated with a skull fracture and possible TBI or traumatic brain injury.

The nose is deformed in several directions; his breathing is irregular and shallow at thirty times a minute. I can hear good air movement on both sides of the chest, which I'm surprised at with the heavy bruising over the right middle chest. The left wrist is shattered with shards of bone exposed and the obvious lower extremity injuries.

He does have a right radial pulse (on the thumb side of the wrist); it's weak at 130 beats a minute. He's pasty pale with cool and clammy skin...*he's in shock.*

The radial pulse is a key finding. Joe gave me this tip many years ago. When assessing a trauma patient, or any patient, feel for a radial pulse first (if they're breathing), this will give a quick clue as to how serious they are, at that moment. The blood pressure needs to be at least in the 80–90 range on the top number to generate a radial pulse. If you cannot feel one, the blood pressure is below this and they're critical.

This is a valuable "trick of the trade."

Rocky has the long spine board ready and helping Steve finish applying the MAST pants.

Steve had to "align" both legs into the correct anatomical positions before the MAST can be applied. It's a gruesome task as the bones grinding together make a sound never easy to hear.

Sam has an oxygen mask over the patient's mouth and nose.

"This is going to have to be the priority when we get into ambulance, Mark, we're barely keeping this airway open," Sam exclaimed.

"Roger that, Sam," I said and nodded.

Once in the back of the ambulance, I applied the rubber tourniquet to the upper right arm and quickly found the vein I would use. The 14 gauge went in and we have IV access. This would be crucial for the next step, securing the airway.

When we have a patient critically injured or unable to protect their airway, we'll administer medications that render them deeply unconscious and paralyzed for several minutes.

We'll then intubate which allows for a higher concentration of oxygen to be given as well as protecting the airway from aspiration or vomiting.

This procedure is called RSI or rapid sequence intubation.

It's not without risk. Once you administer the drugs, the patient will stop breathing. If you cannot secure the endotracheal tube or ventilate them with the bag valve mask, they can have catastrophic outcomes and worst case, die.

I'm very aware of this. My advantage will be having Sam and Dana working together with me, almost instinctively anticipating the next move instead of reacting to it.

Paramedics save lives. EMTs save paramedics. This passage describes Sam and Dana perfectly. Without a strong EMT, it's difficult for the paramedic to provide the advanced critical care for a successful outcome.

Dana has the LifePak 12 hooked up. She'll call out numbers as I am performing the RSI procedure, the heart rate, blood pressure, and SpO2.

"Heart rate 132, blood pressure 84/50, SpO2 at 90%," Dana called out.

"Okay, thanks, Dana, everyone ready?" I called out and made eye contact.

Sam and Dana both nodded affirmatively.

The first drug is etomidate. It quickly puts the patient into a deep anesthesia or sleep.

The second drug is succinylcholine. We call this drug *sux*. It will rapidly bring on muscular paralysis and importantly render the gag reflex in the throat inactive. With this reflex active, we could stimulate vomiting with the laryngoscope blade and create a disaster of an airway. The sux will last for several minutes.

We only use the RSI procedure for patients who are breathing. If they're in cardiac arrest or not breathing, we go straight to intubation as they have no gag reflex.

The patient responds almost immediately to both drugs and lets out a final audible sigh.

With the laryngoscope in my left hand, I carefully insert the curved blade along the split tongue and down his throat in search of the epiglottis, the landmark structure above the vocal cords and trachea. The bright light on the tip of the curved blade has the back of the throat well lit.

I'm not sure who's vying for the best view, me or Sam. She's focused with the suction wand and ensuring my view stays at maximum.

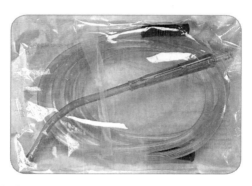

This is the "suction wand" we use to clear the airway of everything from vomit, blood, secretions, and everything else that can stand in our way from securing the airway. The tubing connects the wand to the suction device. We have a strong portable unit as well as a wall mounted one in the medic unit.

I'm at the epiglottis, and the vocal cords come into view along with the tracheal opening. I slide the tube in from the right corner of the mouth and watch it pass into the trachea, and we now have control of the airway.

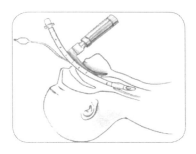

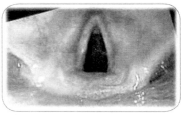

As I get to the epiglottis, the vocal cords are right below it. This is an actual view of what I look for and watch the endotracheal go through the opening a couple inches, into the trachea.

"Okay, Sam, it's all yours now, let me know if that tube moves any at all," I said.

"Roger that," was Sam's usual confident response.

"Hear rate 136, blood pressure 84/50, and SpO2 at 96%," Dana called out.

"Roger that, thanks, Dana," I said.

It's important to repeat the assessment and adjust any treatments if needed. I placed a second dressing over the left neck as the first one is becoming soaked. The bleeding from the ears has slowed. The periorbital ecchymosis has nearly swollen both eyes shut. The bruising over the right chest is becoming more discolored, and we suspect a ruptured liver which needs an OR.

The inflated MAST has stabilized the femur fractures. Steve did not inflate the abdominal section on the MAST. If he did, we could potentially cause greater bleeding into the chest by pushing blood from the pelvis up into the chest area.

Dana splinted the left wrist with bandages and a cardboard split, very effective.

"Looks like being the patient for splinting classes paid off," I said and smiled at Dana.

"Splinting and packaging, *tools of the trade*," she replied, and nodded approvingly as she looked at the splint.

I noticed a vein in the lower right arm and placed a second IV. Dana extracted a drop of blood from the IV catheter for a glucose check or sugar check.

This is indicated for any unconscious patient or anyone with an altered level of consciousness. Just because they have an injury doesn't mean they can't be a diabetic and have a critically low blood sugar.

We use a glucometer which gives us a reading measured as mg/dL, milligrams per deciliter. Normal levels are between 70–110 mg/dL. We just call out the number and all understand what it means.

If it's above 500, the reading comes out as "HI," if it's below 20 the reading comes out as "LO."

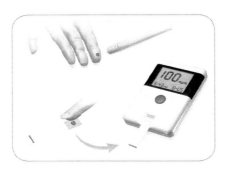

"Blood sugar is 100," Dana announced.

"Roger that," I nodded affirmatively.

We arrived at RGH to a small army of help, security personnel, and ED techs, all welcome in helping us get the patient into suite 12 and awaiting trauma team.

Once into the room, the ED physician, Dr. Stein, took over and the focus shifted toward prioritizing care. It is quickly confirmed the patient needed to go to the OR for a liver laceration.

The liver is a highly vascular organ located in the right upper abdominal region and extends across the front and to the left side. It is vulnerable to blunt or penetrating trauma. The liver is your body's *oil filter*.

His CT scan showed multiple skull fractures but no TBI. This would be monitored closely. The wrist and femur fractures were pinned, and he'd be admitted to the trauma ICU in stable but critical condition.

We spent the next twenty minutes cleaning the medic unit. Steve showed up with the rescue and said the patient's brother came to the scene after we left.

The brother explained the patient called him via cell phone and said he was having engine problems and trying to set down in the field where he crashed when the phone went dead.

We would learn the patient's name is Randy. He's thirty-three years old, married with a five-year-old son and a web designer working out his home. After seventeen days at Regional, Randy was discharged home to recover. He faces months of physical therapy and on last report retired from flying.

Rocky and I made it back to the station at 1400 hours. We're starving and decided lunch would be something you could fix quick, eat fast and be happy with that.

The EMS call gods have no mercy for seeing someone starve even though they're saving lives and ending suffering.

If you need regular meals and time to eat them, EMS probably won't be a good fit.

During our *feasting*, Sandy came into the kitchen, and with a controlled look of frustration said, "Mr. Freeman called again and now wants to know what you did with his dentures, and his remote control is missing."

Rocky covered his mouth to keep from spitting food while beginning to laugh.

I stared at Sandy and halfheartedly considered obtaining legal counsel when we were saved by the tones.

"Rescue 41, Medic 42, respond code three for an unconscious male, possible overdose, 966 Ogden Way, time out 1415 hours."

Rescue 41 was pulling out the bay as Rocky and I made it to the ambulance and followed after them.

Dispatch has updated us this is the Sunshine Retreat, a halfway house for recovering addicts.

We arrived on scene within four minutes. One of the administrators met us out front.

I introduced myself, "Hi there, my name is Mark, and I'm the paramedic in charge, what's going on this afternoon?"

"Hi, Mark, thanks for getting here so quick, one of the residents collapsed in the bathroom and he's turning blue, we think he might have OD'd on heroin," she said.

"That would definitely do it," I said, "We better get in there."

We followed her down the hall and eventually into room 14. The patient is being dragged out the bathroom by two staff LPNs.

He's purple from the neck up and taking an occasional exaggerated deep breath and unresponsive. He has secretions trailing from the right side of his mouth and nose which created an eerie glistening from the overhead lights.

"His roommate heard him collapse and yelled for help, we found him on the floor with the needle hanging out his left arm, purple and not breathing," one of the LPNs explained.

"Okay, good job on getting him out there, where's the needle now?" I asked.

"I put it in the bathroom sink, we didn't see any others," she said.

You always need to be aware of the needles for obvious reasons.

"Great, thanks you guys, Sam, you and Dana take over on the ventilations. Rocky, I'm going to look for an IV site if you want to get an IV set up," I said.

"Roger that," Rocky said.

A quick look for other life-threatening injuries doesn't reveal anything obvious.

Dana used the small towel we keep on the gurney and wiped the secretions from the patient's face, then placed the mask over his mouth and nose and nodded to Sam.

This towel can be worth its weight in gold when trying to establish a critical airway.

With a couple squeezes of the bag, the terrifying blueness throughout his face began to look pink again.

He has the classic pinpoint pupils. They resemble two *periods* in a sentence, the hallmark sign of narcotic influence.

Heroin can be injected, snorted, or smoked. It's an opiate derivative and overdose is manifested by shallow or slow breathing or not breathing at all. The narcotic decreases the drive to breathe, and if they aren't discovered quickly, they will go into cardiac arrest and die.

With heroin being an illegal narcotic, the user never knows how pure his stash might be. The potency can change from dealer to dealer. When they inject what they *believe* to be the amount they are used to, they can quickly go unconscious and stop breathing.

I put a rubber tourniquet above both elbows and didn't see any visible veins popping. You could follow where veins were supposed to be by following the scars and needle marks up and down both arms. On the streets, these are known as track marks.

My fallback site was the neck. The external jugular is usually accessible. Sure enough after gently tipping his head to the left, the right external jugular was quite large, and inviting for a 14 gauge.

This IV site would be used to administer Narcan, and hopefully bring the patient back to the world of the living.

Narcan is a narcotic antagonist which means it reverses the effects of the heroin. The response would be almost immediate with the patient awakening to the sobering reality of seeing everyone around him and realizing this day was not going well for him.

The IV went in smoothly. I secured it by looping the IV tubing over the right upper shoulder and taping it heavily. We need to ensure we have everything planned in case the patient woke and became combative or vomited.

Fighting was an inherent risk with overdoses and unpredictable. This would be secondary to having the high of the drug wiped out by the Narcan and even though you just saved them from certain death, they aren't always in good moods.

Vomiting wasn't uncommon after Narcan administration and could be alarming by being projectile in nature. You can minimize this by administering the Narcan slowly but sometimes it just happens.

Here we go.

Not even half the syringe is injected into the IV port, and he opened his eyes and did the quick scan around the room with the "what happened and what's everyone doing in my room" look.

"Hi there, my name is Mark, I'm a paramedic. Can you hear me?" I asked.

"Yeah, what happened?" he said trying to sound normal like everything was a big misunderstanding.

"Well, we think you might have overdosed," I said.

"Oh, dude, come on, I didn't do anything," he said trying to maintain the protest.

"We need to take you to RGH so they can make sure you're okay," I said.

"Oh please, man, I don't need to go there, I said I didn't do anything," he pleaded.

We continued on this conversation line for several minutes before he eventually began crying and admitted to using just "one time" this afternoon.

It doesn't register to them by even having this conversation is a miracle considering they were minutes or even seconds away from death. If he'd gone unnoticed, it wouldn't have been the same outcome; we'd have found him dead in the bathroom.

During the trip to RGH, I learn the patient's name is Steven. He's twenty-eight years old and has been using heroin since he was fifteen. He's been in prison twice for burglary and released last month after serving two years.

He's on probation and condition of his release was contingent on remaining clean from heroin at the halfway house for six months. There's a very good chance he'll end up back in prison for this episode. It's difficult not to have empathy.

If we could somehow get Steven's story to kids at risk, could we make a difference? We don't seem to have a shortage of users.

The rest of the transport was uneventful. Steven was quiet and withdrawn. We were directed to suite 4 where Sally, one of the nurse's in the ED took the report. Steven was the third heroin overdose of the day in the ED.

Back to the station, and Rocky and I couldn't figure out why we're so hungry, then it dawned on us we haven't eaten much today. We're picking through the fridge and not being too particular when Sandy came back to the kitchen, again.

"You're never going to guess who called," she said.

"Oh no, now what did we forget to put back in place?" I asked.

"Well, Mr. Freeman called and wanted to pass on how grateful he is for everything you guys did for him, he's feeling better and looks forward to the next time he sees you," she said while enjoying our shock.

Rocky stared as if Sandy was speaking some foreign language.

"Are you sure he called the right number? If he calls again could you tell him we were transferred to another station?" I said.

"Nice try," she said.

"He specifically requested you guys for all his transports," she said and then turned and walked out the kitchen with a wide grin.

"Next time…?" Rocky said, and then trailed away lost in thought.

The break over the next several hours provided the time to catch up on reports and get the ambulance back up to par on supplies. We carry enough to go on several calls before restocking but you never want to let it get to that point.

The evening news was covering the ultralight crash, and as soon as they started mentioning the medical part, we were interrupted by the familiar tones.

"Rescue 41, Medic 42, respond code three for an eighty-four-year-old female with chest pain, 104 Simpson Apartment A-Alpha, time out 2214 hours."

Getting the address correct is a crucial part of being able to provide timely medical response and care. Whenever there was a letter involved in the address, dispatch would clarify with a phonetic reference.

In this case "A" could end up sounding like a number or any other confusing words. Hearing the designated "Alpha" after the letter left little doubt.

Traffic is light and the five-minute response was good.

Walking up to the apartment was odd with the porch light being off and no lights on inside the place.

With all us standing in front of the residence, I knocked on the door and waited. After several seconds, we looked at each other and I knocked again, this time a bit harder. I reached down and twisted the doorknob just as a curiosity and thinking we may have to yell into the residence. We could have a patient who may not hear too well or, worst case, may even have collapsed.

The next sound we heard was not what we expected and created an instant fear along with surges of adrenalin. The unmistakable sound of a pump shotgun being racked and angry male screaming out on the other side of the door, "Who the hell is it...I have a gun, and I'll blow your a——s away!" He shouted out clearly and legibly.

"It's EMS...EMS, we got called for chest pains," I managed to yell out meekly while trying to hide behind a 4 × 4 post and become as small as possible.

We hear a chain being taken off the door as the porch light came on and the door slowly opened. The male immediately lowered his intensity and apologized for the drama and scare.

"I've been broken into twice in the last month," he said.

"I didn't call you guys, what address you looking for?" he asked.

"104 Simpson, Apartment A," I said.

About then Steve had dispatch on the radio, and they updated the patient's address is actually 1104 Simpson Apartment A.

We were off by a few blocks.

The patient called 9-1-1 on her cell phone and somehow 1104 became 104. That little missing number nearly turned our night into disaster.

After a quick apology from our end as well as firm handshakes, we retreated to the vehicles and drove to 1104 Simpson. This time, the front door was open and patient is standing in the doorway waving to us.

I walked up and introduced myself, "Good evening, my name is Mark, I'm a paramedic, and you did call us, didn't you?"

"Yes I did…my chest…is hurting…and I'm having… trouble breathing," she said with the noted pauses between sentences.

When you hear a patient speaking in shortened sentences, this is a significant red flag. Especially when it's accompanied by chest pain, she could be having a myocardial infarction or heart attack.

We assisted her to a chair in the living room where everyone began getting equipment set up.

Sam placed an oxygen mask over her mouth and nose, Dana was getting the LifePak 12 hooked up, Rocky was getting an IV bag *spiked* or setup, and Steve was bringing the gurney through the door.

"So can you tell me your name?" I asked.

"Mabel," she said.

"Okay, Mabel, when did this start and where's your pain?" I asked.

"It started…about thirty minutes ago when I was getting ready for bed," she said.

"The pain is right here," she said as she's pointing to the entire right side of her chest.

"It's heavy…and I…I can't seem to breathe," she said and then a pause to catch a breath.

Dana handed me the 12-lead EKG strip. This is a more in-depth look at all parts of the heart and diagnostic for myocardial infarction.

The 12-lead gives us twelve different views of the heart. From the top, the bottom, the sides, the middle, the big picture. It can show us irritability or actual ongoing muscle death, a heart attack. It's quick to obtain, we'll place six patches across the chest, one on each limb (wrists and ankles) and the LifePak 12 will provide two additional virtual views to give us the "12 lead."

My heart sunk when I looked at printed strip. Mabel is having a significant heart attack. She's also having a heart attack that's difficult to treat with our standard drugs.

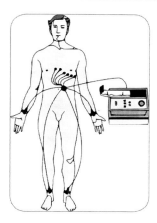

A common drug we use with cardiac-related pain is nitroglycerin.

Nitro has the properties to enlarge the vessels of the heart (coronary arteries) which in turn deliver more oxygen to the parts of the heart needing oxygen and thus relieves some of the pain.

It's given in spray form under the tongue or sometimes as a quick-dissolving tablet also placed under the tongue. It has an inherent secondary side effect of lowering the blood pressure. When we see a heart attack like Mabel is having, we'll be extremely cautious with the administration.

"Blood pressure 184/110," Dana called out.

This would allow us to give at least one spray of the nitro with relative safety.

After getting the IV established and reviewing everything, we're ready to transport. We're in a time critical mode as definitive treatment cannot begin until arrival at the hospital. Every minute can count and affect the outcome.

The saying in the prehospital arena is, "Time is muscle."

The quicker we get the patient to the hospital, the more heart muscle tissue potentially saved.

Blood pressure has come down to 134/88 after one spray of nitro. This means we cannot give any more. This is too much of a drop from the baseline; the next spray could put her in critical readings.

RGH has been alerted and we are declaring this as a *cardiac alert*.

This puts Mabel at the center of attention along with a *reservation* for an immediate evaluation in the ED. She may be a candidate for some type of procedure to reopen the blocked areas and minimize the damage to the heart.

We handed Mabel off to the cardiac team at RGH with all our information and treatments.

As we were getting the ambulance back together, we had a critique of the call outside the ED.

Everyone thought it went very well minus the address mix-up. Sam and Steve were the only ones to leap off the porch and take cover at the sound of the racked shotgun.

Steve was a military police officer in the army, and with his extensive training, it was an instinctive move. Sam, being the resident firearms expert, made it second nature upon hearing the familiar sound.

Before we left the hospital, we had an update that Mabel was off to the coronary catheter lab, and they were going to insert stents, the artificial mesh devices that keep the coronary artery open and hopefully restore circulation to the affected areas and limit the damage that could occur.

It's just another one of our typical days in EMS, no two ever the same, just the way we like it.

3

PARTY ON

THE START OF a three-day weekend with sunny weather and a payday isn't a good combination for folks in EMS. The vast majority of the public will enjoy the time with a safe, uneventful, family-oriented, and personally satisfying weekend. For others, it can have terrible outcomes.

Rocky and I completed our daily rig inspection and equipment check and ready for whatever the day brings. Sam and Dana also finished their daily routines on the rescue.

Steve walked into the truck bay and said he had a surprise for us and requested we all move into the dayroom.

Our dayroom is our place to relax around the station. We have recliners arranged in a semicircle around a big flat-screen TV. The biggest problem we generally have is who gets the remote, and they decide what we watch which no one usually agrees on.

Steve is on one knee in front of the TV and reading the back of a DVD case.

Sam walked over and reading it over his shoulder, *"Keep Your Patient Safe When You Unload Your Gurney."*

"Did you order this on *purpose?*" she asked.

Dana chuckled and reclined her chair fully flat pretending to snore.

Steve turned, looked at both of them with his finger up as if to make a point and was squelched by the tones coming from the ceiling speakers.

Our much-anticipated training would be put on hold.

"Rescue 41, Medic 42, respond code three for a possible DOA, 4200 Oaks Park Road, Apt. 17, time out 0832 hours."

Both units quickly went en route. We should be there in less than four minutes. We're monitoring scanner traffic and police will be on scene before us.

A DOA means dead on arrival. It can be natural or traumatic in nature. We will respond code three, lights and siren as there have been instances where the person was not actually dead and still viable.

We arrived at the front entrance to the complex, stopping at the large legend board with locations of apartments. Apartment 17 is in the back, we have to navigate incredibly large speed humps to get to it. We literally had to crawl over these humps in fear of destroying the undercarriage of the medic unit.

"How can an average car make it over one of these things," Rocky said with a hint of frustration.

"They probably park outside the complex and walk in, quicker," I reasoned.

There are two police cars parked in the lane of travel, and we pulled up behind them. After grabbing all the gear, we make it to Apt. 17.

Walking into the apartment was an immediate challenge to the visual and olfactory senses.

"Blanket curtains" are strung above the windows allowing odd streaks of light into the room. The warm beer and stale cigarette aroma along with personal BO and rotting food thicken the air.

Sam and Dana have "raised cheeks with squinty eyes and scrunched nose" facial expressions. I think we all do now that I look around.

Two police officers are talking to a male in his twenties sitting on the couch with an obvious hangover.

He's disheveled with puffy eyes that are heavily bloodshot, visible even in the darkened room, wearing boxers and a T-shirt, sitting on the edge of the couch leaning forward, rocking back and forth, and mumbling something none of us can understand.

One of the officers acknowledges us with a nod and points to the kitchen.

As we enter the kitchen, the cause of the friend's anxiety becomes dramatically obvious.

His roommate is DOA, lying face up on the floor next to the fridge.

He also looks to be in his early twenties, has dried vomit in and around his eyes, packed in both nostrils and pooled in his wide-open mouth.

There's a massive and gaping open laceration to the center of his forehead which resulted in heavy discoloration and swelling. The bleeding from this has created a deep pool surrounding his head on the floor and is coagulated and crusted.

It's a horrific and graphic sight reflective of a violent end.

We also notice blood on the corner of the counter and a small crumpled throw rug tangled next to his feet.

This was obviously a very tragic accident in the fact it looks like he came into the kitchen and fell after getting tangled with the throw rug, struck his head on the counter, and in an unconscious state aspirated and died.

He's cold to the touch and rigor has set in, he's been dead for several hours. There's nothing we can do for him.

I walk around the corner toward the roommate; he looks up at me with anticipation and momentary hope and asks, "Is he all right, man?"

"Well, there isn't an easy way to say it, but I'm afraid not, he died several hours ago from what we can determine," I explained trying to be honest and not offer any false hope.

"Oh man, oh man, oh man," he starts chanting and puts his head back into his hands.

After letting this sink in for almost a minute, I need to get a little more information for the patient care report I have to complete back at the station.

"Can you tell me anything that might help us figure out what happened?" I asked with no intent.

He quickly looked up and with a serious tone said, "Oh no-no-no, you're not going to pin this on me, man, I didn't have anything to do with it."

I reached out and put my hand on his right shoulder.

"Hey, I don't for one second mean that, I just wondered if he was drinking or had any medical issues," I explained.

"We got hammered last night, isn't it kind of obvious, I woke up and went to get some juice and found him freakin' dead man, he's my...was my best friend," he said.

"Seriously, do we have to talk about this now, man? I really can't think," he added while almost hyperventilating.

"Okay...is there anything we can do for you?" I asked.

He shook his head and just kept rocking with his head in his hands. I looked at the officer and nodded good-bye, he did the same.

"What a tough way to start the day. Wake up and find your best friend and roommate dead," Rocky said as he navigated the speed humps on the way out the complex.

"No doubt," I said, "No doubt indeed."

Back at the station and I got the paperwork completed for the DOA. One thing we never seem to have a lack of and that's paperwork. Our reports are done electronically which expedites the process. On the average, it can take twenty to thirty minutes to complete a patient care report depending on the complexity of the situation and treatment administered. The patient care form becomes part of a person's medical history for years and then I'm not sure it ever completely goes away.

It's important your report has no opinions, only facts. It takes months and even years to develop your style. And then it can still be ostracized by a good lawyer.

Oftentimes we're called to court it's generally as a witness for the prosecution, and your report will be part of the presentation. If you have spelling errors and incorrect information, it can be humiliating, and potentially disastrous for the case. Good defense lawyers will go to any lengths to discredit your testimony.

We *are* experts in being qualified to chart what we see, as in a patient assessment.

Write what you see, let the reader make the determination.

It's embarrassing to be asked to describe your expertise in ballistics or blood alcohol assessment certification when you chart things like, "Patient was very drunk" or "Patient was shot multiple times" or "Patient was very drunk and shot multiple times."

No opinions!

Another poor choice of words in a patient care form is "appears." This word means you don't know.

When the chart has statements like, "Patient *appears* to be acutely short of breath," someone might question if you were with the patient at the time.

You can end up sounding silly with this word.

If instead you wrote, "On arrival, patient is leaning forward on the couch with *tachypneic*-fast respirations, *circumoral cyanosis*-blue around the lips, and speaking in one and two-word sentences," the reader will look at this and say, "This person is having acute difficulty breathing."

You certainly wouldn't chart something like, "Patient *appears* to be decapitated."

So writing what you see will keep you out of trouble *and* from getting those dreaded "see me" notes from the medical program director.

The afternoon is spent reviewing protocols. As prehospital care providers, we're not independent practitioners. We have a set of protocols or treatment care guidelines we follow for every scenario we respond to.

Of course we can't remember the last call that fit the treatment guidelines exactly; nothing is ever black and white. That's probably the genesis for the KISS theory which is a universal term throughout EMS, "Keep It Simple Stupid."

Don't overcomplicate things, they aren't that hard.

We're able to practice under the license of a medical program director or physician advisor, and our director is Dr. Gary Stein, an emergency physician from RGH.

Dr. Stein meets with the crews regularly and reviews our medical documentation for compliancy as part of a QA or quality assurance audit. He's incredibly supportive of the EMS program and we're fortunate to have him for a director.

He's empathetic to the challenges we face in EMS and will occasionally ride as a third on the ambulance. It's exciting for him to get out the ED and see firsthand what we do prior to getting the patient to him in the controlled confines of the ED.

As usual, once you start something around the station, the tones will interrupt it, and there they go.

"Rescue 41, Medic 42, respond code three for an unconscious male after a fight, 605 Edwards St., The Foxx Hole Lounge, time out 1822 hours."

The Foxx Hole Lounge is popular with the under thirties crowd. We've had many calls here. A few months ago, we transported a female who nearly died with alcohol poisoning. She was celebrating her twenty-first birthday and was as close to being her last as she could get.

She was found in the bathroom, unconscious and aspirated and severe lung problems. She spent a month in the ICU and fortunate to not only survive but also have no permanent deficits.

As we pull into the parking lot, there are three patrol cars at the side entrance. An officer is waving us to the door.

"Hi guys, you got a male subject beaten pretty bad, he's unconscious. We're still working the scene but he needs you guys pretty quick," he explained.

"All right, we'll take care of him," I said as we grabbed our kits and headed through the door.

The patient is lying on the floor in the back corner near the bathrooms. He's on his left side with a large pool of blood surrounding his head. He's unresponsive to voice or taps to the shoulder. The blood is coming from multiple lacerations to the face and head, mouth, and nose. The left eye is swollen shut with a deep purple ring, periorbital ecchymosis.

Witnesses would report seeing the patient fighting briefly with another male. He took a punch to the side of the head which immediately dropped him. He was then kicked repeatedly in the face before bystanders pulled him away. The patient has been unconscious since hitting the floor.

Dana is holding the head in-line with regard to cervical immobilization as we prepare to roll him onto the long spine board.

The facial injuries are extensive. There's a large gaping laceration over the left brow; the left upper lip has a full-thickness laceration extending up and through the left nostril along with several missing teeth. There is also a small trickle of blood coming from the left ear canal.

With the bleeding from the mouth, he's gasping and choking. Sam has the suction unit and clearing the airway which is ongoing.

"Mark, this airway isn't getting any better," Sam commented.

"Yeah, I noticed that, Sam, we better expedite things here," I replied.

Steve is cutting clothing away and things just became exponentially more critical.

There's a two-inch penetrating wound to the left upper chest with bubbling during each breath. This is a sucking chest wound.

This is a classic example of why we cut clothing off. We cannot "see" what's beneath the clothing.

Steve places his gloved hand over the wound.

A sucking chest wound needs immediate coverage. Left open it interferes with oxygen exchange and can lead to severe and fatal hypoxia (low oxygen state). It's also known as an open pneumothorax.

This scene may have just become an attempted homicide or even end up as a murder case.

Rocky placed an occlusive dressing over the chest wound which seals the opening.

I can feel a radial pulse at 120 beats a minute. His skin is pale, cool, and clammy, in shock.

Suddenly, four males watching us are moving closer. One of them makes a comment about the patient getting what he deserved and suggesting we not work too hard to help him.

He then starts directing personal comments to Sam and Dana, and this scene is spiraling out of control.

Two of the officers stand between us and the four who aren't backing down.

In the next second, three more officers come through the front door and control has shifted back to the officers.

We're using this opportunity to get the patient out the door and into the ambulance and headed to RGH.

"I'm going to get this IV and let's get set up for the RSI," I told Sam and Dana.

The both nodded affirmatively.

Dana has the LifePak 12 hooked up and calling out numbers.

"Heart rate 116, blood pressure 76/44, SpO2 88%," she said.

I have the drugs drawn up for the RSI procedure. Dana pushed the etomidate and then the sux. The drugs worked quickly and patient is ready for the intubation.

As I slid the laryngoscope blade into the back of his throat, I'm met with thick clots of coagulated blood and just as I got a view of the vocal cords the back of the throat filled with blood.

Sam is trying to provide suction but the clots are thick and difficult to manage.

"Heart rate dropping, SpO2 is 82%," Dana called out with urgency.

I have about five seconds to get this view cleared and tube passed.

Miraculously, Sam moved a clot with the suction wand and I have the view I need.

The tube passed into the trachea, Sam connected the bag valve and squeezed in a breath. We see the chest rise and let out a collective sigh.

This was an intense fifty seconds we didn't need.

"Heart rate back to 120, SpO2 is 92%, blood pressure 80/48," Dana called out.

"Roger that," I said shaking my head side to side.

With two minutes before arrival to RGH we have to reassess.

The right pupil is still reactive. The chest seal is working as intended and holding. I can feel the rice krispies under the skin all around the stab wound, but no evidence of tension in the chest building.

The alcohol aroma is heavy in the back of the ambulance. This is almost a given with any assault of this nature. There is one common denominator in violence, alcohol.

From unloading the gurney to going into suite 12, the trauma team sprang into action with mesmerizing efficiency.

The chest tube is placed in the left side and quickly fills with blood. Then to CT (computerized axial tomography) CAT scan for the head assessment. He has an epidural hematoma on the left side of the head which is bleeding in the brain and requires immediate surgery.

The epidural space is a layer beneath the skull, and a hematoma is a collection of blood. This qualifies as a TBI or traumatic brain injury.

There are multiple facial fractures, and he will have a permanent vision loss in the left eye.

His alcohol level is .24, three times the legal limit.

The patient's name is Taylor. He's thirty-one years old. This afternoon he was brutally assaulted and left for dead. He will survive this incident but live with the consequences the rest of his life. There was no arrest made and the investigation remains open.

I'm driving to the station for the start of the shift, and it's a beautiful morning, the sky is blue, it has the makings of a perfect day. I notice a few people driving in a hurry, changing in and out of lanes like they're in a race, aggressively tailgating, and then realize where I am going, to the station and maybe seeing some of them later today.

I put my stuff away and made it into the truck bay. Rocky, Sam, and Dana have started the morning vehicle checks.

"There are some crazy drivers out there this morning," Rocky commented as he closed the hood on the ambulance.

"Oh, you saw them too," I said in agreement.

"Yeah, I was only frightened for my life twice, once when Sam cut me off pulling in to the parking lot," Rocky said.

"Hey, you were driving too slowly, so I went around you," Sam countered.

This had the makings of a great debate on who was the slowest and fastest when the tones decided it was a draw.

"Engine 61, Rescue 41, Medic 42, respond code three for motor vehicle crash, possible DOA, approximately the 4200 block of Christian Valley Road, time out 0846."

This response was on the border we share with District 6. We have a mutual aid agreement with them along with a solid working relationship. Their captain is Willie Neeves, a strong leader and experienced EMT. He sports a traditional handlebar moustache, thick and always perfectly groomed.

This response would take us nine minutes.

When a car crash is dispatched as a possible DOA, something significant has taken place. We may arrive and find the injuries aren't as severe as the caller thought, or it could be exactly as dispatched.

We respond with an open mind and believe we can make a difference.

"Engine 61, Rescue 41, Medic 42, be advised county deputy on scene confirming the location, also advising two patients, one confirmed DOA, the other is unconscious, needing extrication, continue code three response."

Steve and I both received the update as did Capt. Neeves.

Christian Valley Road has a speed limit of 45 mph. It's a two-lane windy road with shallow embankments and large trees on both sides. We've responded to crashes on this road over the years, and driven recklessly, it can be a deadly stretch.

However, if you're driving the speed limit and paying attention, it's like any other road.

We see a county patrol car ahead with its overhead lights on. Engine 61 has arrived from the opposite direction and stretching hose lines and preparing extrication equipment.

Rocky put the medic unit in position to make an exit and not get blocked by any other arriving units.

As we exit the ambulance, the smell of gasoline from the crashed car and exhaust fumes from the extrication power unit permeate the air.

The crashed vehicle is over a small embankment and smashed into a large tree. It struck the tree head on with the majority of the impact on the passenger half of the car. There are no skid marks prior to where the vehicle left the road.

The DOA patient looks to be in his late teens. He's heavily entombed around twisted metal in what used to be the passenger compartment. The only view we have of him is parts of his upper body and head. He has no carotid pulse and is ghostly pale. Considering the massive injuries to his head, chest, and abdomen, he likely died on impact. There's a heavy alcohol aroma emanating from his side of the vehicle.

The driver also looks to be very young. He's unconscious and unresponsive, pinned grotesquely with the steering wheel flat against his chest and metal crumpled around him.

As we get a better view of his entrapment, the steering wheel actually splintered and impaled into his chest just over the right clavicle (collarbone) and base of his neck. There's approximately three inches protruding from the chest, and it's difficult to tell how much is impaled or what structures it affected or direction it went after entering the chest.

He's bleeding from his nose, both ears, and making deliberate gasps with periods of no breathing. This is a graphic and perilous presentation given the position he's in. There's a strong alcohol aroma coming from his side of the car.

The Engine 61 crew make short work of popping the door and now the delicate task of spreading the car's frame to gain access to him. The vehicle will not give up its hold on him easily.

Dana made her way onto the hood and managed to fit into the smallest spaces, crouched next to the patient. She positioned his airway and for now, he's taking more regular breaths. She also has an oxygen mask next to his face.

This is a move only someone as small and strong as Dana could pull off.

A firefighter from District 6 has a large tarp shielding her, and the patient from the Jaws of Life activity going just inches from them.

The car is shuddering with pieces of steel popping and slowly yielding as the Jaws of Life gets us closer to extricating him from his metallic prison.

Capt. Neeves and I are discussing the plan for getting the patient out.

"I think we'll be ready to move him in just a few minutes," Capt. Neeves advised me.

"Okay, Cap, we're ready on our end," I said.

Rocky is in the medic unit preparing equipment. At the least, we'll need to secure the airway, establish IV access, and monitor the cardiac status. Every minute is precious when you have a critically injured patient.

Sam is next to the car with the long spine board waiting to place it at the opening being created.

Dana looked at me and simulated an intubation motion several times from atop the car.

I nodded to her and gave the okay sign. Rocky would get things ready on his end.

Steve is standing by with dressings to secure the chest from the impaled steering wheel portion.

Suddenly, the final piece of the car is breached, and we have free access to our patient. Dana is continuing to hold his head in line as Sam places the board next to his seat. He's easily pivoted and secured onto the long spine board and headed to the ambulance.

He's ghostly pale and still having the breathing irregularities. I place a tourniquet on each arm above the elbow.

Rocky has us headed to RGH. We're on scene for eighteen minutes, an eternity in EMS trauma time.

Sam and Dana are providing breaths with the bag valve mask.

I finish cutting the clothing and start a quick assessment. The impaled piece of wheel is solidly implanted and bleeding around it is minimal. Whatever it has done, it also sealed itself off.

There are no breath sounds on the right side and rice krispies throughout the entire right chest. I grab the big needle and place it between the second and third ribs, midclavicular. Air can be heard for several seconds followed by oozing blood.

The pelvis is sunken on the right side and looks like a fracture to the right lower leg. The leg fracture will be a low priority.

The pelvis injury is significant; he could bleed to death from this injury by itself.

I have the LifePak 12 hooked up and the first readings are dire.

"Heart rate at 140, blood pressure 54/32, SpO2 isn't reading," I called out.

I notice a large vein on the left midarm and put a 14 gauge into it. With the RSI drugs prepared by Rocky while setting up the ambulance, I switch places with Dana and ready for the intubation.

She pushes the drugs and we see immediate results. With Sam operating the suction, I have a clear view of the cords and watch the tube pass into the trachea.

We're now two minutes from RGH. Sam is ventilating with the bag valve, Dana splinted the right lower leg with a cardboard splint and then looked at the LifePak 12.

"Heart rate 142, blood pressure 50/30, SpO2 not reading, glucose 104," she called out as she extracted a drop of blood from the IV needle.

"Okay, Dana, good call on the glucose, thanks," I said.

We're arriving at RGH where security and two ED techs are waiting. They open the backdoors as Rocky is stopping the medic unit.

We cautiously make it to suite 12 where it seems like every nurse and doctor in the hospital is in the room working feverishly to stabilize this young kid.

Heart rate alarms suddenly start chiming loudly from the EKG monitor on the wall and one of the nurses yelled out, "He just coded."

Coded is terminology for cardiac arrest.

I walked out the room, and Rocky, Dana, and Sam followed me out to the ambulance. We sat down on the curb. Seeing a person this critically injured takes a toll, the body is so fragile, and difficult to survive an insult like this.

Steve pulled up in the Rescue and walked over and sat with us.

"Not good I take it?" Steve asked.

"We gave him a chance, that's about it," I said.

Brenda, the ED supervisor came out to let us know they stopped the efforts. She said the trauma surgeon commented about the heroic efforts that took place and getting him here with a pulse was some kind of miracle.

We thanked her, cleaned the ambulance, and went back to the station.

We would learn the patient's name was Theo; he was twenty years old and engaged to be married next month. His passenger was his cousin; Bryce, he was eighteen years old and going to be the best man at the wedding. In a single incident, families would forever be changed.

It's hard to make sense of scenes where the incident was probably 100 percent preventable. How was the decision made to ignore the warnings of driving while under the influence? The consequences of poor choices can have catastrophic outcomes.

Last year, we responded to a head-on collision that killed a seventeen-year-old teenage girl and sixty-four-year-old woman. Several witnesses following the seventeen-year-female report she had been weaving in and out of the lane of travel and driving at irregular speeds.

She then abruptly drove directly into the path of the oncoming sixty-four-year-old female who was in a small compact vehicle. There was zero time to react and collision was instantly fatal for both occupants.

The investigation concluded the seventeen-year-old was texting her boyfriend for several minutes right before the collision.

When I was going through paramedic school, we went through defensive driving training. Our instructor was of the opinion there was no such thing as an accident.

"All collisions or crashes are preventable," he would say.

It's difficult to argue with that philosophy.

4

DR. STEIN

DR. GARY STEIN has been in meetings here at Station 4 since 0800. Joe, Capt. Neeves, and two other training officers from neighboring stations get together quarterly to evaluate our patient care guidelines.

Our protocols get this frequent review and adjustments as needed based on trends in medicine, requirements for specific response areas, and keeping all treatments current with national standards.

We enjoy a liberal system and have freedom to employ some very aggressive treatments all under the watchful and supportive direction of Dr. Stein, our EMS boss.

After the meeting with the training officers, he's conducting our monthly run review with the crew where he goes over select cases and discusses what went good and sometimes, what didn't. It's a learning tool and not to be looked at as a punitive session.

After ninety minutes, we've finished and got our usual very high marks for compliancy and appropriate treatment decisions.

Dr. Stein likes to say, "When you work with good folks you get good results."

He will also occasionally ride along to watch us "do what we do." Of course, he isn't ever with us when we do our most exciting work.

Today that would change.

We're in the day room and having an informal discussion about life in general, and Sam seems to be getting most of the attention with the recent spotlight she's had in periodicals about her firearms expertise and marksmanship. She's rapidly becoming highly nationally recognized.

"Sam, you have to take me to the range and get me better with my pistols," Dr. Stein said.

"Well, I have the afternoon reserved there tomorrow, no time like the present," she said with a wry smile.

In the next second, the tones resonated through the ceiling speaker.

"Rescue 41, Medic 42, respond code three at the request of Engine 61, standby for an occupied structure fire, 6700 Eagle Creek Road, time out 0955 hours."

I looked at Dr. Stein and said, "Want to come along?"

With a youthlike grin he nodded and said, "Let's go."

Both rigs pulled out with lights flashing and sirens blaring and we're off.

This response would take about six minutes, a straight shot up the freeway. Engine 61 had closer ambulances but they were on calls.

We're still a couple minutes out and could see the foreboding smoke column in the distance.

Suddenly we got a chilling update from dispatch.

"Rescue 41, Medic 42, Engine 61 advises they have one patient, a male, unconscious and with burns to the face, chest, and legs."

Steve and I both received the update.

I looked back at Dr. Stein and said, "Looks like another chart for the review."

He nodded affirmatively and said, "Well, let me know what you need me to do, this is your scene."

Several fire units along with two county deputy patrol cars are parked along the side of the road leading to the residence. As usual, Rocky is able to position the medic unit where we won't get blocked in.

As we park, Capt. Neeves is walking up to the ambulance.

"We're going to have to stop meeting like this, good to see you guys again," as he nodded to Dr. Stein and me, "We got a guy burned pretty bad, the crews are ventilating him with the BVM, he's over here," Capt. Neeves explained.

"Okay, we'll take care of him," I said and grabbed the airway kit and followed him with the crew and Dr. Stein next to me.

Capt. Neeves looked at Dr. Stein with a grin and said, "So the chart review was that bad you had to follow him, huh?"

"Paramedics!" he said and then winked.

Walking toward the house is like a scene out of an action movie.

The deafening roar of the fire with angry flames dancing wildly seeming to extend a hundred feet into the air, the sound of the structure cracking and buckling as it's on the verge of collapsing, smoke billowing in clouds so thick they block out the sun, water being sprayed in vain attempts to gain the upper hand, heroes in action.

It's hypnotic, hard not to stare with awe but the radiant heat is uncomfortable even from this distance and we have a more urgent calling.

We locate the patient behind one of the fire engines.

He's supine (face up) and being treated by two EMT firefighters. One of them has the BV mask sealed over the patient's mouth and nose, the other is squeezing the bag providing rescue breaths. They're both drenched with sweat, faces dirty, and wear looks of steel determination.

The patient has suffered extensive burns with skin peeling and sloughing away from the chest, abdomen, and tops of both legs. His face is blackened with eyebrows and hair burned off leaving patches of red skin, the lips are swollen and nearly twice their normal size.

The priority will be securing his airway before it becomes too swollen from the burns and also address pain control. Even though the patient is unresponsive, he can still be experiencing pain.

The firefighter squeezing the bag valve quickly gave us the information they knew.

"This is Oscar. He's sixty-five years old, a neighbor called 9-1-1 after the fire vented through the roof. They knew Oscar was home. We arrived and the initial attack crew found him a few feet inside the front door. He's been unresponsive since they brought him out," he explained.

"Okay, thanks you guys, great job. Sam, you and Dana take over for them so they can get back to the scene, Rocky, get us ready to get out of here, Steve, let's get this airway handled," I ordered.

I looked at Oscar's face. In that instance, I had a little voice in my head *screaming* at me to do a quick look with the laryngoscope.

I didn't hesitate.

I reached into my airway kit and set an endotracheal tube cross Oscar's chest.

I attached a laryngoscope blade to the handle and gently slid it down Oscar's throat. This would likely be the only attempt we'd have at securing the airway with oral intubation.

If it didn't work, he'd almost certainly need a surgical opening of his neck, a cricothyrotomy.

The moment cannot get any tenser. Dr. Stein is standing directly behind me basically getting the same view I am.

The burns and swelling inside the mouth are extensive, the tongue is engorged. It's worse as I get toward the back of the throat. All of the sudden, I have a perfect view of the vocal cords; I see swelling around them that could seal his airway within seconds.

With my right hand, I grabbed the tube off his chest and slid it down his throat watching it go through the opening to the trachea. I withdrew the blade and held onto the tube for Oscar's life and let out a sigh.

"Great job," Dr. Stein said, "I was ready for the cricothyrotomy."

A cricothyrotomy is a surgical opening to the neck going directly into the trachea. It's a quick alternative for a patient whose airway cannot be established or controlled by other means. It's also a very invasive procedure and can be more complicated that it sounds.

"We didn't want to break our perfect record of never needing one," I said with a bit of pride.

Sam now has the bag valve attached to the end of the tube and providing breaths.

Dana is cutting the rest of Oscar's clothing which is difficult with much of it burned into his skin.

Rocky has the gurney ready and two burn sheets opened. He'll lay one on the gurney and the other to cover Oscar.

The burn sheets are large blue sterile sheets that basically provide a bit more sterility than a regular sheet. In reality, it's difficult to create a true "sterile field" in the prehospital arena.

Dr. Stein was right there helping us lift Oscar onto the gurney. We're in the ambulance and headed out with a seven-minute scene time.

Dr. Stein put a stethoscope to his ears and listened to the chest as Sam was squeezing the bag valve.

With the burns, it was difficult to see chest rise and fall.

"I hear a lot of wheezing but they sound equal, great job you guys, I'm impressed," he said.

Dana managed to get the LifePak 12 hooked up by putting the electrodes on parts of the chest with minimal burns.

"Heart rate 136, blood pressure 160/120 and SpO2 at 91%," she called out.

"Roger that," I said.

I look at Oscar's left arm, and he has the largest vein just above the wrist. I took advantage of this and put a 14 gauge into it.

Dana took the needle to get blood for the glucometer and announced, "Glucose is 106."

"Roger that, 106," I repeated.

Dr. Stein recommended we administer etomidate and sux to ensure Oscar didn't wake and start fighting with the tube in his throat before we arrived at the emergency department.

We also administered morphine for pain control.

During the reassessment, there are extensive second and third-degree burns to most of the legs, the lower abdomen through the chest and most of his head.

He could easily be approaching the 50 percent to 70 percent range, and these carry very high mortality rates. Along with the significant burns and associated burnt skin smell, we can't help but notice the nearly overpowering alcohol aroma mixed in as well.

Two of the major contributors associated with house fire-related injuries and deaths are alcohol and nonworking smoke detectors. Oscar has at least one of them.

We arrived at RGH and had the usual incredible response from not only the trauma team but also the burn unit team as well. Dr. Stein drew strange looks from the staff as he walked in with us looking and smelling like one of the crew. Today, he was one of our crew and we're happy to have him.

"You guys did a fantastic job out there, I couldn't help but feel I was in the way, I think I'll stay here in the nice controlled confines of the ED," he said and then shook all our hands.

"You're welcome with us anytime, and we're happy to stay in our little world out here," I said.

Oscar was being prepped to go to the OR and then to the burn unit. His blood alcohol level is 0.33 on arrival, over four times the legal limit. Would this happen being sober? Who knows, it couldn't have made things worse!

Over the next couple weeks, we followed Oscar's progress every other day. He's still intubated, and in a medically induced coma on a ventilator.

His road to recovery will be the toughest of his life. He still has many weeks, maybe months before they can hope to see improvement.

He lives alone and has two daughters that live out the area. They've come to stay by his side during these difficult days. He'll need all their support if he hopes to have any chance of moving forward.

Fire investigation determined the fire started in the kitchen, at the stove. They believe Oscar may had started cooking and passed out, awakening after being burned and collapsing near the doorway where he was found.

We rarely go late into the afternoon without having a call. Today we've had just that, no calls. Rocky went into the truck bay several times just to be sure the ambulance hadn't left without him. When you're used to going from call to call, the lull can be disquieting.

We wouldn't enjoy this respite too often and were about to go from zero to a hundred and become part of a life or death struggle with the sound of the tones.

"Rescue 41, Medic 42, respond code three for a fourteen-year-old male with breathing difficulties at the Central Gate Mall food court, time out 1630 hours."

We're out the door quickly and should have a three-minute response. The mall would be crowded this time of day and traffic heavy.

"Rescue 41, Medic 42, be advised the caller says the patient is getting worse, possible allergy to peanuts and having an allergic reaction."

Steve and I both acknowledged the update. If this was a true allergic reaction, time could be critical in playing a role for a successful outcome.

When someone is having an allergic reaction that progresses to anaphylactic shock, the body starts shutting down quickly. The upper airway tissues around the tracheal opening can swell, closing it off, the smaller airways in the lungs become constricted, the blood pressure drops, and death can be seconds away.

The EpiPen can break this vicious cycle if administered quickly after the reaction begins. People with known severe allergic reactions will carry one of these kits. They are about the size of a large cigar and administered to the lateral thigh, right through clothing. The epinephrine (adrenaline—same thing) is injected automatically and the response can be lifesaving.

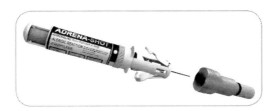

This is an example of what the EpiPen might look like. There are several brands and styles people carry. It is designed to be quickly employed, remove the cap, and press against the outside of the thigh where the needle goes through the clothing and into the leg and automatically injected.

We arrive and park in front of the food court entrance, a mall security officer is waving us. He quickly walks up to my side of the ambulance as I am getting out.

"Hi guys, we got a pretty serious kid here, I think he's having an anaphylactic reaction," he said with concern in his voice.

"Okay, lead the way, we'll follow you," I said.

The mall is crowded as anticipated. Our presence created immediate interest with people following and staring with natural curiosity.

In the food court area, we find the patient lying on the floor next to a table, arms outstretched and desperately trying to get a breath.

His friends are on both sides of him watching helplessly as he struggles second to second with this life-and-death drama.

"Karman, Karman, they're here man, hold on, Karman," the one friend shouted.

"He's allergic to peanuts and ate a peanut cookie," the other friend said.

"Has he used an EpiPen or does he have one?" I asked.

"He left it at home," they said nearly in unison.

Karman's face is swollen with eyes nearly shut, his tongue is protruding, and lips are swollen. He's a range of colors between bright red and deep purple. The sounds coming from his mouth are high pitched or stridor, an indication he's very close to losing his airway. He has no radial pulse (wrist) and is unresponsive to my calling his name.

Stridor is a terrible presentation for an airway.

Think of letting the air out of a balloon and stretching it side to side, restricting it, the loud high-pitched sound is exactly what is going on here, an airway swelling shut.

Sam's immediately at his head with the bag valve mask and oxygen. Dana is trying to make a seal over his face. Steve's cutting Karman's shirt off and has the LifePak 12 hooked up.

Rocky has the kit open and drawing up epinephrine and hands me the syringe.

I quickly insert the needle into Karman's left arm and push the plunger administering the medication.

Sam and Dana are struggling with getting air in.

That's when Steve calls out, "He just coded, Mark!"

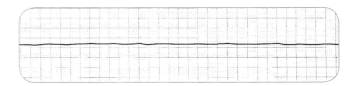

This is asystole, or flatline, no cardiac activity. We DO NOT shock this rhythm as there is nothing to shock.

I looked at the monitor just in time to see the last beat going across the screen and then asystole which is flatline and my heart sank.

Karman just *died* on us.

Steve was instantly in position and began compressions. I hear a collective gasp go through the large crowd that has amassed.

Strangely, I'm only aware of our little area and pressure to get this boy's heart beating.

Rocky tossed me a rubber tourniquet as I slapped Karman's right arm several times looking for a vein. I was able to get a 16 gauge into it. After plugging the IV tubing into it I'm running it wide open, trying to "fill the tank."

"Another box of epi," I said with my hand out in front of Rocky.

He already had the box open and I quickly had it going through the IV line.

"Are you getting any air in?" I asked Sam.

She nodded and said, "Yeah, now we are, and it seems to be getting a little easier."

"Okay, we're going to check the rhythm here in a second, Dana, you and Steve switch places when we do," I said.

"All right let's stop, still asystole, flatline, go ahead, and continue compressions, Dana," I said.

I was getting ready to push another epi when Karman's hand came up grabbing Dana's hand while she was getting ready to deliver the second compression.

We got him back, I thought and feeling a wave of relief, now I have to keep him that way.

"He's taking full breaths and fighting us on the mask," Sam called out.

"Sounds good, Sam, let's switch to an oxygen mask," I said.

Karman was taking full clear breaths. The swelling to his lips was subsiding and we could actually see his eyes. His color is looking more normal, the red and purple is fading quickly.

"Heart rate 140, blood pressure 96/60," Steve called out.

"Roger that," I said.

"Go ahead and run that whole bag in, Rocky, then hang another bag and slow the drip," I said.

Rocky nodded while staring at the bag that was just about to run out.

Karman got a small round of applause from the crowd and that's when I actually looked up, and there are at least a hundred people standing intently watching us.

Karman slowly opened his eyes and was looking around.

I leaned close to his ear, "Can you hear me, Karman?" I asked.

He nodded without saying anything.

"Well, my name is Mark, I'm a paramedic and we're going to take you to the hospital. It's very important to just relax and let me know if I can do anything, okay?" I said.

He nodded again and this time looked me face to face.

We got Karman secured on the gurney and out to the ambulance. On the way to RGH, he continued to improve.

His blood pressure stabilized and heart rate would stay high because of all the epi I put in the IV line, plus the initial dose in the arm.

I gave him Benadryl through the IV which will help with the hives that are also part of the allergic reaction. The hives are raised red welts and can be itchy.

By the time we got to RGH, Karman was talking with a normal voice and able to answer questions.

His main complaint at this time is being cold and jittery from the epi and chest is sore from Steve and Dana's compressions. He'll be evaluated for this and to ensure he doesn't have a rib fracture.

His mother came into the ED frantic. Her last report from his friends was he died at the mall after having the allergic reaction.

There are few words that can describe the moment she saw him lying on the hospital gurney, smiling at her as she rushed to his side, followed by the mother and son embrace, and uncontrolled tears of happiness.

I don't think he'll forget his EpiPen anytime soon. I have a feeling his mother will somehow attach it to him, permanently.

Each year, the state EMS office sponsors a two-day EMS conference. This is one of the first years we're off duty and it's being held in a city two hours from here. Sam, Dana, Brandon, and I are planning on attending and very excited.

Steve and Rocky have plans and it's their loss. Joe will be part of the educational staff and with another group.

When we can head out of town and not hear tones or answer calls, we'll take full advantage of this opportunity.

The conference is set up with EMS vendors along with an impressive lineup of continuing education classes that will nearly satisfy the rest of our requirements toward our upcoming recertification.

As with any conference away from home, there are events that go on that aren't part of the venue, these are probably better left as hard lessons and classic memories learned.

We're back on shift after the three-day whirlwind adventure and moving a little slower than normal.

Rocky commented, "You guys are all strangely silent, anything go on at the conference? Have a good time? Anything you want to tell me?" he asked to no one in particular.

The bay is silent, Sam, Dana, and I are acting as if he isn't speaking to any of us.

"Oh, okay, I get it, you guys went out and had fun without the 'Rock,' okay, no problem, I understand," he conceded.

I looked at Dana and Sam as we shared a grin. Brandon was in the day room, in a fully reclined position with a *Medical Terminology* book open, across his chest with snores coming from above.

The rigs all look good, and we finished just in time for the first call of the day with the tones sounding a *little louder* than usual.

"Rescue 41, Medic 42, respond and stage for an unknown type problem, my partner is taking the call now, she is getting information relayed from MHP, 1001 Rhodes Ave., and time out is 0855 hours."

Both units are quickly headed that way.

"Mental Health Professional, huh," Rocky said.

"Yeah, sounds intriguing," I said.

We're just a couple minutes from where we planned on staging when dispatch gave us the important update.

"Rescue 41, Medic 42, you are clear into the scene, you have a twenty-two-year-old male, he has ingested a razor blade and Mental Health on scene with law enforcement, 0900."

By now, we don't try to rationalize why people do what they do in their delusional and acute psychotic states. Our goal is be respectful to the patient, provide the highest quality of care, and get them to the next level without judgment.

We arrived and parked next to a police car. There's one other police unit on scene and a white county vehicle with a placard on the door: MHP Services.

A smartly dressed female is coming out the house and walks up to my side of the ambulance. She has a look of concern and holds her right hand out as I step out and close the door.

"Hi there, I'm Patricia, the lead MHP, thanks for coming. We have a very tough case here," she said while lightly shaking my hand.

"Hello, Patricia, my name is Mark. I'm a paramedic and this is my crew, how can we help this morning?' I asked.

She took a deep breath and sighed heavily.

"I have Blaine, he's twenty-two, and we know him quite well. He has a very complex psychiatric history involving ingestions," she started.

"Yeah, we heard something about a razor blade," I said.

She took another breath and exhaled again before speaking.

"More like five hundred of them," she said as I stared at her unable to process this number and thinking I may have misheard her.

"I'm sorry, did you say *five hundred*?" I asked while beginning to understand her unease.

"Yes, five hundred, he admitted to it, and one thing we know about him, he's very honest. We found twenty packages with twenty-five razors in each, they're all empty," she explained.

"He told me he started eating them last night at midnight and called this morning to report it after getting frightened," she said.

"He'll be cooperative and shouldn't be a problem. I've called RGH, they're expecting him," she added as we walked toward the front door.

Blaine is sitting at the dining table with one of the officers standing next to him. He's pasty pale and his color has my immediate attention.

He has cuts with dried blood around his mouth, cuts to both hands with dried blood, and has a very distant and empty look I don't think I've ever seen…it's almost painful to see.

Where do we start?

I knelt down next to him and introduced myself.

"Hi, Blaine, my name is Mark, I'm a paramedic. This is my crew. Sounds like we're going to give you a ride to Regional this morning," I said and gave him a reassuring pat to the shoulder and then checked a radial pulse.

None!

He slowly turned and looked me in the eye.

"I'm sorry, I'm so sorry, please, I'm sorry," he said and a single tear ran down the left side of his face.

"Oh, Blaine, trust me my friend, we'll do anything we can for you," and put my hand on the back of his shoulder giving him a couple light squeezes and pats.

I wasn't sure I understood it but I had a strange empathy for Blaine. He presented with an almost childlike innocence, and I want to do whatever I can for him.

His skin is cold, clammy, and his fingernail beds are white.

I have a very uneasy feeling about Blaine's presentation.

Sam, Dana, and Steve got him secured in a flat position and headed to the ambulance. I notice he has beads of sweat on his forehead and lips have lost their color.

I can see Sam, Dana, Steve, and Rocky are also very aware of how critical he's presenting.

I stopped and briefly spoke to Patricia, "I think he's a very sick kid right now and may have something going on internally," I explained.

Patricia stared at me intently, "Do you think he'll be okay?" she asked.

"Well, we're going to do everything we can, we'll know more at Regional," I said.

"Okay, I'll meet you guys there, I have to stop at the office," she said.

As I walked toward the front door, Steve met me with a concerned look, "He's starting to throw up, it's all blood and razor bloods," he said.

I got into the back of the ambulance, Dana has a large basin and holding it near Blaine's mouth, it's half full with clumps of bright red blood and hundreds of pieces of razor blades, and he's now unresponsive.

His color just went to ghostly pale.

"Let's get moving, Rocky, code three," I called out.

We felt the rig accelerate and would have a five-minute transport to RGH.

Dana is working the suction, and Sam has the bag valve mask over Blaine's mouth and nose. Blood is spraying around the mask piece.

I'm cutting clothing and quickly applied the patches for the LifePak 12. I moved to the jump seat to secure the airway.

"Dana, get an IV setup, and put the tourniquets on for me," I said.

"Roger that," Dana said and started working.

"Okay, Sam, let's see what we got here," I said as I introduced the curved laryngoscope blade into Blaine's mouth.

"Suction," I said.

Sam is face to face with me vying for space and offering suction as she can.

"Heart rate 154, blood pressure isn't reading, SpO2 isn't reading," Dana called out.

"See any IV sites?" I asked as I was looking down Blaine's throat.

"I think so, it's ready when you are," Dana said.

"There they are, hand me the tube, Sam," I said.

I watched the tip of the tube go through the vocal cords and into the trachea. Sam is now ventilating with the bag valve.

"Heart rate is slowing; 50-40-30-20-he's coded!" Dana called out.

"No, Blaine, don't do this to us, hang on," I whispered aloud.

Dana braced her knee against the gurney and began chest compressions.

I found the IV site Dana saw and somehow put a 14 gauge into it, the IV bag is running wide open.

"We're asystole, flatline, keep going, Dana," I said.

I looked at Blaine's expression as Sam was ventilating him and strangely it looked the same as it did in the house.

We arrived at RGH and had plenty of help on the ramp. Dana stood on the side frame of the gurney continuing compressions as we went into suite 12.

Dr. Stein took over care. The room was eerily silent as I explained the circumstances. When I mentioned the five hundred razor blades, everyone had empathetic looks for this very troubled young man.

Twenty-six minutes after we arrived, Dr. Stein called the efforts. Blaine was dead.

As we're cleaning the ambulance, Patricia came walking up.

"Sorry it took so long, phone calls, how is he?" she asked.

I looked at her and just stared, didn't know what to say.

"Oh no, you're not serious?" she asked.

It was obvious Patricia had a working relationship with Blaine and shocked by the news.

We went back to the station and Sandy was waiting in the truck bays.

"I was just informed you guys have a tour coming in, a field trip from a day care center. They'll be here in thirty minutes," she said, "Sorry for warning time."

"That's okay, Sandy, maybe we need to see some silly screaming kids," I said.

That's exactly what we got.

5

BIG DECISIONS

THIS HAS BEEN like old home week at station 4. Eric Wright has a temporary assignment back with Rescue 41. Dana has the next few shifts off and planning on going to Las Vegas for a pediatric conference.

Eric was the third member on Rescue 41 for almost three years with Steve and Sam. One day out of the blue, Eric shocked all us by announcing he wanted to take the step to paramedic. As strong a member of our team as he was, we encouraged his desire as we would for any member of the team wanting to climb another rung on their personal EMS ladder.

After completing paramedic school, he faced another difficult decision in transferring away from Station 4 to an opening on an (Advanced Life Support) ALS ambulance at a neighboring station. It was however a very intelligent move in fostering his new role as a paramedic.

We miss having Eric as part of the team, and his absence certainly left a hollowness that Dana filled quite amazingly.

Sam still likes to tell Eric we got the better end of the deal from it all.

Our station sponsored the location for an Advanced Cardiac Life Support (ACLS) class to be held over two days, Friday and Saturday. Eric and I are both ACLS instructors but cannot be part of the dedicated staff since we're on duty Friday.

ACLS is a certification all advanced life support providers, paramedics, intermediate level EMTs, doctors, nurses, respiratory therapists, pharmacists, and many other in-hospital staff are required to be current with. It covers the algorithms which is basically the *suggested treatment guidelines* for cardiac emergencies from chest pain to full cardiac arrest and strokes. It follows a decision tree approach until you can get the patient to a higher level of care. This is a two-day, sixteen-hour class divided between lecture and practical stations that simulate a cardiac scenario. It's mandatory to be updated every two years.

Today, Friday, we're available to help out where needed, but as EMS goes, the calls start early out of the chute with those familiar tones.

"Rescue 41, Medic 42, respond code three for a forty-two-year-old male subject complaining of chest pain, he's in a vehicle on the side of the road on County Road 4 at mile post 3, time out 0818."

It's not uncommon to get calls for people pulled over on the side of the road. Sometimes they might be talking on the phone with their heads down or reading maps or even taking naps. We call them slumpers and occasionally it turns out to be an actual emergency.

"Rescue 41 and Medic 42, be advised this patient is in a tractor-trailer rig, he is semiconscious, pale and sweaty, there are several bystanders attempting to get him out the vehicle."

Steve and I both acknowledged the update and this added a twist I suddenly had a bad feeling about.

We arrived to see people waving us to their location next to the cab of the big rig. The patient didn't pull completely onto the shoulder, and we'd need to claim the entire right lane.

For added safety, Steve positioned Rescue 41 about a car length behind the medic unit. State patrol units were also arriving, and this has now become a very large scene and about to become larger.

The patient is sitting in the cab of the tractor-trailer which has him over six feet off the ground. He's every bit of 450 pounds, and as I tap his leg trying to get his attention, I hear snoring respirations that sound agonal in nature. In other words, he's in cardiac arrest.

Agonal respirations are ineffective breaths which do not produce a normal respiratory effort. They're common after a patient goes into cardiac arrest.

I looked at Steve and said, "He's coded, we need to get him out of there, now."

Steve looked at me and said, "Got a plan?"

I didn't and could feel each second agonizingly ticking by. We had the very real potential for serious injury letting him fall the distance from the cab to the pavement.

Could this get any worse? I thought.

I called Rocky, Eric, Steve, and two of the troopers over to the opening of the cab and hastily said, "Let's start pulling him out and supporting as we go, it's not going to be pretty but we need him out, now!"

We initially couldn't get his massive frame moving. However, once he began to come our way, things progressed rather quickly, and he came out fast landing heavily on top all us.

During this *controlled exit* from the cab, we could hear several shocked gasps from the bystanders as he flattened us.

Somehow, I was able to keep his head from smashing to the pavement and ended up on my backside with his head in my lap. Eric's legs are sticking out from underneath the patient's belly, Steve is tangled in his enormous legs, and Rocky has both arms under there somewhere.

During this removal, Rocky caught a boot to the right eye which is rapidly swelling and becoming blue. He's going to have periorbital ecchymosis, a black eye.

The two troopers are trying to untangle us. After a little maneuvering, we're all free and have the patient on his back, in the lane of travel.

Steve quickly began chest compressions. Sam and Eric initiated ventilations with the bag valve mask.

I start cutting clothing from the waist up, and the first thing I noticed was a well-healed zipper.

This is a surgical scar along the midline of the chest indicating he's had open-chest surgery and gives us information he could have a cardiac history, despite his young age of forty-two.

Working around Steve's compressions, I got the fast patches placed, and LifePak 12 hooked up and ready to look at the EKG rhythm after two minutes of CPR.

With the current ACLS guidelines, treatments for cardiac arrest revolved around two-minute increments of CPR with the overall goal of minimizing hands off the chest time.

"Okay, everyone, after this set of compressions, let's stop, and see what we've got. Rocky, you take over for Steve," I said.

"Roger that," Rocky and Steve chanted.

"V-fib," I called out, "We'll shock at 200…everyone clear," and the energy was delivered as Rocky immediately resumed CPR.

The shock elicited another collective groan from the bystanders.

Watching cardiac arrest resuscitation can be traumatizing for bystanders to witness. With the fast and deep chest compressions and defibrillations, it certainly isn't something you see every day.

I found a good IV site at the middle of the left arm and put a 14 gauge into it. Steve handed me the IV bag Rocky setup, and we now have IV access for drugs.

Steve extracted a drop of blood from the IV catheter and called out, "Blood sugar 110."

I nodded affirmatively to Steve and told Eric he might as well get the patient intubated while he was up at the head.

This would be a tough intubation with the large heavy head, small mouth opening, and almost no neck. Eric would need all his experience for this to be successful. There's no such thing as routine in EMS, if you get complacent, you invite disaster.

We're nearing the end of the two minutes of Rocky's compression.

"At the end of this round of compressions, we'll check the rhythm again, Rocky, you and Steve switch again," I said.

"Okay let's stop and check, V-fib, let's shock at 300, clear," and the shock is delivered.

Once again on cue, the collective gasp from the crowd.

Steve resumed CPR, Eric was ready for the intubation attempt, and Sam standing by with the suction. At the same time, I gave epinephrine through the IV line.

Holding the laryngoscope handle in his left hand, Eric inserted the long blade down the patient's throat. From the onset it was a struggle, just not enough room to get a good view.

Finally, after a few seconds, he called out, "I can see the cords, hand me the tube please, Sam."

With a careful and deliberate insertion of the tube, he pulled the blade out the mouth, and let out a long exhaustive breath.

"It's good," he said, "I saw it go through the cords."

With my stethoscope in my ears and listening to several areas over the front of the chest, I can hear clear and equal breath sounds. Eric made a difficult intubation look easy, it was a great job.

"Sounds good right there, let's get it secured so we don't have to do that again," I cautioned everyone.

"Roger that," Eric added.

I happened to notice, it looked like the patient was moving his right arm each time Steve compressed the chest.

"Hey everyone, I think we may have something here," I said, "Steve, stop compressions and let's check the rhythm."

We not only have a pulse back, but also we have a good-looking EKG rhythm on the LifePak 12 screen.

We're getting a blood pressure reading of 136/66, heart rate is 124, SpO2 at 94%. It's early but we're heading in the right direction.

Now we have to get him packaged on the long spine board and loaded into the ambulance. This will be a feat in itself. With everyone working together, we managed to get him secured and headed to the hospital.

During the transport, we review everything and make sure we haven't missed something.

After a thorough head-to-toe assessment, everything looks good and vitals are remaining stable.

I yelled to the front of the ambulance, "How's the eye, Rocky? Can you see okay?"

"Oh sure, as long as I don't have to look too far to the right," he said.

I could see his face in the rearview mirror, his right eye is all but swollen shut, not to mention colorful.

We arrived at RGH and appreciated the reception party on the ramp of the ED.

Dr. Stein took over care and everyone was entertained at the story I gave on how we ended up getting him out the big rig and still managed to have a favorable outcome on scene.

Rocky couldn't figure out why everyone who looked at him did a double take as we came into the ED. It wasn't until he went into the bathroom and fully realized what a frightful sight he was and had quite a shiner forming beneath the eye. He was happy Rachel wasn't on duty at the time.

We later learned the patient's name is Charley. He's forty-two years old; lives with his invalid mother; and between him and his sister provide total care for her. It was hard not feel a deep empathy for their situation.

Charley was admitted to the (Coronary Care Unit) CCU after having stents placed in two coronary arteries. He would be discharged to home after seven days in the hospital.

Back at the station, the ACLS group was on a break and all interested in the case. We took a few minutes after their break to go over the call. Explaining the extrication was the highlight as they expected the ACLS part to go as planned.

Rocky was the show and tell for verification it was indeed as tough as it sounded.

Rachel came to the station for lunch and brought the kids. Hank and Abby were intrigued with Rocky's shiner. Kelsey was more interested in something stuck between a recliner cushion in the day room. The kids were part of the family here and made themselves quite at home.

Rachel was getting ready to leave and we couldn't find Hank. We looked through the truck bays, the day room, and the kitchen and finally Sam called us down the hall to the bedrooms. We have small individual rooms for each crew member.

Hank is curled up in the smallest ball, nuzzled into Rocky's pillow on top his bed. He's sleeping so soundly, snoring, and isn't aware of us all standing in the doorway watching him, snickering. After a few minutes, he opens an eye, and the very tip of his tail starts wagging.

"Come on, we have to go home and get you guys some food, let's go," Rachel said and slapped her thigh once.

The afternoon class was about to start and the tones ensured Eric and I would not get to be part of the class.

After hearing the dispatch, the ACLS class should have just come with us today.

"Rescue 41, Medic 42, respond code three for a fifty-six-year-old male with chest pain, 206 Industry Way, The Lumber & Builders Warehouse, time out 1314 hours."

The Lumber & Builders Warehouse was a five-minute response. Traffic is fairly light after the noon-hour rush.

As we're arriving, there are two workers out front waving and pointing to the side of the building. There's a door where another employee is standing and waving. The workers from out front followed us and met me as I opened the ambulance door.

"Thanks for getting here so quick, we got a guy who's hurting pretty bad, he's having chest pain like a heart attack or something, his name is Gerry," he said.

"Okay, we're getting our stuff and we'll follow you," I said.

Walking into an office area of the building; several people have chosen to remain at a distance with worried looks.

When people want nothing to do with someone hurting, it generally means things are bad.

The patient is sitting on a chair leaning forward holding his chest. There's a female and another coworker standing on either side of him. They also have concerned looks.

The patient is pasty pale, sweating profusely; breathing rapidly, his hands and fingernail beds are white and has a look of doom across his face.

Gerry could be a training poster for, "What do you look like when you're having a massive heart attack."

"Hi there, my name is Mark, I'm a paramedic, what's the main problem right now?" I asked.

"Pain, my chest, I don't feel good," was Gerry's response.

"We're going to help you, Gerry, just hang in there," I said.

Gerry gave a small nod and is looking worse by the second. I check Gerry's radial pulse and it's absent, his skin is ice cold.

"When did this start?" I asked.

"About half an hour ago, I thought it would go away," he said.

Steve removed Gerry's shirt by pulling it up and over his head. Eric has an oxygen mask over his mouth and nose.

Sam is getting the LifePak 12 hooked up and has to dry the chest before applying the electrodes from the profuse sweating.

Rocky has the kit open and getting an IV setup as Eric applied the rubber tourniquet to Gerry's left upper arm.

Sam finishes the 12-lead EKG and hands me the printout. He's having a myocardial infarction, a heart attack at this very second, and he won't get better until we get him to the cardiac team at RGH.

Gerry is still being supported by his coworkers when he began leaning heavily to his right, then took a deep gasp and went unconscious into cardiac arrest.

The female coworker screamed out and put her hand over her mouth, other employees stared in disbelief.

Steve and Eric got Gerry to the floor.

The LifePak 12 is showing ventricular fibrillation. When we see it happen, we can go straight to a shock before performing CPR which is what I did.

"Sam, charge to 200," I ordered.

The high-pitched whine of energy building in the LifePak 12 was deafening in the silence of the small room as the coworkers stared with fright.

"Clear," I said and pushed the button on the front of the monitor, and Gerry arched to the energy.

The rhythm changed back to a regular pattern with a good carotid pulse. I took out my pen and put the trademark 'X' over the left carotid.

Gerry opened his eyes, blinked a few times, and asks, "What happened?"

"Well, things just got a bit more complicated for a few seconds," I said. (Sounds better than saying, "Well, you just died for a couple seconds.")

Eric put a 16 gauge IV into Gerry's left arm.

"Heart rate 84, blood pressure 84/44, SpO2 88%," Sam called out.

"Roger that, let's get him on the gurney and get moving," I said.

As Steve and Rocky are lifting Gerry onto the gurney, one of the coworkers comes over to me and asks, "Is he going to be okay? I need to call his wife," he explained.

"Well, as you can probably figure out he's pretty sick right now. I can't tell you more than that at this point," I said.

"Just let her know we'll be at Regional and taking good care of him," I added.

In reality, Gerry could go either way. We need to get him to the cardiac team at RGH for his best chance at surviving this event.

In the ambulance, Gerry looked up and said, "How's my heart? I really don't want to die today, my wife would be upset with me," he said with an attempt at gallantry.

With an agreeing look, I said, "Well, we don't want that to happen either, my friend, she'd be upset with us too. Hang in there, and we'll be at the hospital in just a few minutes."

He looked at Sam, and she offered a reassuring nod and smile.

We got to RGH and the cardiac team took over as Gerry was off to the cath lab. He will recover fully and go back to his family and eventually, back to work.

Before we left the ED, Sarah, one of the nurses, called me over to the desk as she was charting notes about Gerry.

"Hey, Mark, I meant to thank-you for those 'X' marks you guys put on the pulses for us. It really makes things go quicker here, we don't see it too often. In fact, the only time we see it is when you guys come in here. Actually, Eric does it too now that I think about it," she said.

"Well, thanks, Sarah, Eric, and I owe this practice to Joe, one of many tips that shaped both of us to the medics we are today," I said with pride.

Of all the tips Joe has given me over the years, this is one of my favorites. Not only does it make it easy to find the pulse in a hurry, but also, as Sarah explained, the ED appreciates it as they also can assess the patient quickly.

When I have a new EMT ride with us, one of the tasks I have them do is to mark all the pulses they can find on each patient we see, carotids (neck), brachials (upper arms), radials (wrists), dorsalis pedus (top of the foot), and the posterior tibial (inside the ankle).

I was on a call with the District 6 crew a few months back, and one of the EMTs came to me before we left the scene. He told me he never forgot that lesson, and to this day, he checks pulses on every patient he sees.

Very cool!

We came on duty this morning, and the day began as it does every shift: vehicle inspection, equipment checks, and cleaning. It probably isn't noticed too often when we're treating an injured or ill person, but there's a lot of personal pride that goes into making sure our equipment is clean and professional looking.

Rocky and I believe we have *the sharpest* gurney in the county. We put the pillow and sheets on perfectly measured, and no wrinkles. The seat belts are fastened and all set exactly the same with a signature loop over each buckle created with the excess strap.

Rocky loaded the gurney back into Medic 42 when Sandy advised us she had a patient at the front counter in the lobby.

An auto parts delivery driver stopped at the station while having an asthma attack. We transported her and since then, breathing difficulties seem to be the theme for the day.

From asthma, emphysema, more asthma, and a clerk at a convenience store that hyperventilated after a car crashed into one of the gas pumps. There was no damage but it upset her so badly, we transported her secondarily to not being able to calm her on the scene.

We finished dinner, and surprisingly had a few hours to relax and as usual not find anything worth watching on TV. With the day being so busy and everything coming to a screeching halt, we knew it would be a matter of time before we paid a price for the respite.

As the tones go off, we're headed to the bay listening for the nature of the call, and then exchanging glances as if we could have guessed what it would be.

"Rescue 41, Medic 42, respond code three for a thirty-six-year-old male with breathing difficulties, 104 Bates Road, time out 2118 hours."

Bates Road is about six minutes from here and traffic is light. As we turn onto Bates Road, we immediately see a small teenage boy standing in the front yard of the residence frantically waving to us.

As Rocky parks in front of the residence, the boy runs up to my side of the ambulance and opens my door.

"Please hurry, please hurry," he's crying out and near hysterical, "It's my dad, he can't breathe, please hurry, please hurry, my dad," and starts running back toward the house.

As he gets close to the front door, he screams out, "They're here, I told them."

We have all our equipment and make our way to the front door. Next to it is an extra-wide wheelchair ramp. This is never a good sign.

As we walk in, we hear panicked screams coming from down the hall, "Breathe, Alan, oh dear God, please, Alan."

We proceed down the hall and walk into the bathroom. A female is kneeling next to Alan nervously shaking him.

A nightmare of a scenario is taking place.

We're estimating Alan weighs in excess of four hundred pounds. He's naked and lying face up in front of a walk-in shower with an oversized chair sitting in it. The floor is wet as if he just exited the shower.

He's deeply purple, and almost black in color from anoxia, no oxygen. His eyes are open and desperately trying to take a breath without success.

Eric and Sam immediately have the bag valve mask in position over Alan's face.

It's made exponentially more difficult as Alan has a full beard. He also has a small mouth opening with almost no chin. This is one of the most difficult airways you can encounter.

We would quickly learn the female is his wife.

"When did he start getting like this?" I asked.

"He finished his shower and couldn't get out. He slipped and I couldn't straighten his head, and then he started getting purple. My son and I managed to get him rolled to where his head was straight but he just can't get enough air," she said and started crying with her hands shaking and covering her mouth.

The teenage son is standing at the bathroom door; eyes welled with tears, shaking uncontrollably, watching in horror as his father struggles for his life.

We're fortunate the bathroom is large enough to where we have room to work. I asked his wife to step out which gave us a bit more room to maneuver.

Eric is working as hard to keep the seal over Alan's face and only a few breaths are making it in. Alan is now unconscious and eyes no longer open. He still has a carotid pulse. I'm not sure for how long though.

I have an idea I've used only once, but we have to try something different than the current plan.

I'm going to have Steve and Rocky pull Alan up into a sitting position while Eric pushes from the back and hold him there.

Then I'm going to try to intubate him from a standing-over-the-top-of-him position.

The theory is all the weight around his face and throat will naturally drop downward by gravity and potentially make it easier to get the airway secured.

Sam will be in charge of holding Alan's massive head in the correct position. Everyone will have to move quickly and hold their respective positions for several seconds.

I'm ready with the intubation equipment and after a quick review of roles, we're all set.

We'll only have seconds at best before Alan goes into cardiac arrest from hypoxia (lack of oxygen). If he gets to that point, we may not be able to revive him.

Rocky and Steve are in place and each grab one of Alan's arms. Eric is pushing from Alan's back as they get him moving toward sitting. We're using the tub to brace Alan's feet to keep him from sliding forward.

The struggle is epic as Alan slowly moves up. Sam is holding his head from falling backward. Everyone's muscles are struggling almost immediately.

"Tip his head back just a bit, like he's sniffing," I directed Sam.

I'm in position standing directly behind Alan and above his head. I insert the laryngoscope blade into his small mouth. He's not fighting it which is crucial at this point. I make it to the back of his throat and can see the epiglottis, and with a bit of manipulation, I can see the vocal cords below it.

I grabbed the tube I placed on the tub without moving my eyes. At this point, my left hand is shaking while holding the laryngoscope and have only seconds left before I lose my grip. I slide the tube into Alan's mouth, and I watch it go through the vocal cords.

"Okay, let's get him down, slowly, slowly, Sam, get ready to start bagging him," I called out.

Sam has the bag valve hooked up to the end of the tube and squeezing the bag. Alan is so large we cannot see his chest rise and fall but we quickly notice his color starting to change. The deep purple across his face and lips is starting to become pink after several squeezes of the bag.

"Eric, try to find an IV site, and we'll give him something to keep from waking up," I said.

Since we have the airway under control, we want to keep it that way until we get to the ED where they can wake him in a more controlled setting.

"Steve, if you can figure out how we're going to get out here, we should be ready in just a few minutes," I said.

"Roger that, already working on it," Steve said calmly.

"I think I can get this vein in the back of the hand," Eric said.

And a few seconds later, the IV was in. I will use the RSI drugs, kind of in reverse order, but we need Alan not to wake up and start fighting the tube in his throat. If that were to happen, we'd back to square one and at this point, we have no second chances.

Steve came into the bathroom with a medium-sized area rug. By rolling Alan one way and then the other, we have the rug positioned under him. Sam and I are each lifting one of his legs. Eric, Steve, and Rocky are pulling the rug, and we're moving down the hallway and to the front room.

MARK MOSIER

We have the gurney lowered, and after quickly changing positions, one of us on each corner of the rug, we lift it just high enough for Sam to slide the gurney under him.

We now have to lift him one final time to get the gurney raised. The efforts are nothing short of monumental.

I am updating Alan's wife and son with his condition and trying to reassure them as the crew gets him slowly to the ambulance.

"As you can see, we're breathing for him. I put him asleep so he wouldn't be uncomfortable with the tube in his throat. We'll know more after we get to the hospital," I explained to them.

"Thank you for helping him," his wife said and then tightly embraced her son while softly whispering something into his ear.

I'm keenly aware of their fear of almost losing him; this is a husband and father, a family.

"We'll keep working very hard and do everything we can for him," I told them, walked out the door, got into the ambulance, and headed to RGH.

A flashing gets my attention as I look out the side window; the overhead emergency lights are creating rapid patterns off the houses as we drive away from Alan's home. Do people wonder what we're doing at this time of night creating these images onto their windows?

We're still breathing for Alan, and his purple color has changed to a very alive-looking pink.

Eric has the LifePak 12 hooked up and has the first readings.

"Heart rate 114, blood pressure 136/96, SpO2 94%," he called out.

We had to wrap the blood pressure cuff over his lower arm above the wrist as it won't fit around his oversized upper arm. With everything he has gone through to this point, the numbers aren't bad.

It's time to review everything and conduct another assessment. The endotracheal tube is exactly where it was originally placed. His pupils are equal and reactive, a very positive sign. We still cannot see the chest rise and fall, but I can hear air going in with my stethoscope when Sam squeezes the bag.

His wife informed me his last weight was 466 pounds as of yesterday.

I called ahead to RGH and requested additional personnel to meet us on arrival.

Alan spent forty-five minutes in the ED before being admitted to the ICU on a ventilator. He'll be weaned off it through the night. At this point, there's optimism for a complete recovery.

We visited with his wife and son in the family room before we left the ED. We got more of the story about how his epoch struggle began with a simple slip in the shower, when you're as large as he is; oxygen stores are used up more quickly. It was a terrifying experience for them to endure.

Tonight, Alan was a very lucky man, he will go back home to his family.

6

BACK TO SCHOOL

ERIC'S MEDIC UNIT went back in service, and he returned to his paramedic position. It was good having him back here at Station 4 for the last few shifts. He's become an excellent paramedic and no doubt stems from his time spent with Joe and the rest of the crews at Station 4.

Dana is back and claims she wasn't distracted by the allure in Las Vegas. Sam has the most dumbfounded look after hearing this.

"Are we talking about *the Las Vegas*, and talking about *you*, Dana?" Sam said with a slight hint of exaggeration mixed with astonishment.

Dana's cheeks quickly got rosy red, and with all of us staring at her, she finally said, "Well, I may have had some time in between lectures, and at night, and in the morning before classes, and before I left for the airport if you must know everything."

Suddenly, the pedestrian door from the offices opened and Brad Kellen walked through.

Brad is a Station 4 EMT volunteer, and he's riding with Rocky and I today for experience.

As we walked to meet Brad halfway, Sam walked alongside Dana with her right arm around her shoulder whispering into her ear which brought another set of rosy cheeks along with a guilty smile. Guess that will stay with them.

"Good to see you, Brad," I said and shook his hand followed by the rest of the crew following suit.

"Thanks guys, and thanks for letting me hang out with you today, I want to run some calls," he said.

"Oh don't worry, I don't think you'll be disappointed," I said.

The start of the shift is in full swing and busy with essential vehicle checks, equipment inspection, and we're quickly ready for the day.

Brad is asking Rocky questions about some of the equipment and talking about scenarios, and it doesn't take long for those familiar tones to start our day.

"Rescue 41, Medic 41, respond code three to Bryant High School, fifteen-year-old male with severed fingers in the shop class, 1415 Maple Ave, time out 0850."

Our departure from the station is quick, traffic is light, and we'll have a five to six-minute response.

"Do they even still have shop class?" Rocky pondered aloud.

"I never thought about that, can't imagine why they wouldn't," I said and then started wondering the same thing.

Dispatch interrupted the conversation, "Rescue 41, Medic 42, be advised you have two additional patients, both unconscious at this time."

Steve and I acknowledged the update.

I requested a second medic unit in the event we had to transport all three patients. Looks like we wouldn't be able to get rid of Eric as easy as we thought, his medic unit was the next closest ambulance.

We made it to the school in six minutes and a school security officer walked up to Rocky's window.

"Morning guys, it's been a busy start here today and now this…if you go around the back, it's building 7. There will be someone there to guide you in," he said.

"Sounds great, and just letting you know, there'll be another medic unit coming," Rocky advised him.

He nodded and gave a salute as we drove toward the back.

We quickly found building 7, and a female waving us to the main door. We parked and she came to my side of the ambulance.

"Hi guys, thanks for getting here so quick, we have a student who cut three of his fingers off on the table saw. Before Mr. Walters could clear the class, a couple students passed out. We have them lying down with their legs up. Mr. Walters and our nurse are helping Sergio, the kid with the fingers," she said.

"And there's blood everywhere," she added.

"Okay, sounds like we have our hands full, we have a second ambulance coming, they'll be here in a few minutes," I said.

She smiled and pointed to the shop class door.

We entered the room and met with the ubiquitous smell of cut wood. Too bad it wasn't under better circumstances.

It resembles a small battlefield triage area with two students lying on the floor; their legs elevated on chairs and blood trailing from a table saw to where Sergio is sitting a few feet away.

Rocky, Brad, and I went to Sergio, while Steve stopped at the first passed out student, and Sam and Dana went to the other one.

Sergio is sitting in a chair with his head tipped back against the wall. He's holding his left hand with his right hand and has a large dressing over it. There's a fair amount of blood seeping through the dressing. He's pale with beads of sweat on his forehead. Mr. Walters and school nurse are at his side.

"Hi, Sergio, my name is Mark, I'm a paramedic. This is Rocky and Brad, what happened this morning?" I asked as Rocky was opening our main kit.

With his eyes closed Sergio said, "I made a stupid mistake and cut my fingers off."

"Okay, Sergio. Well, I'm going to check your hand out. I need you to take some breaths and hang in there. It may hurt a little, but I won't do anything big unless I tell you first, okay?" I said.

"Uh-huh," he said cringing with anticipation, pain and fear mixed.

He opened his eyes and tried to get a glimpse of the hand as I started removing his bandage but positioned myself in a way that blocked his view.

This is a trick you learn early on after letting a patient inadvertently see their injury which can have deleterious side effects like them passing out or make it difficult to continue treatment from the increased anxiety level. They'll see it soon enough, preferably in a more controlled venue than here.

As I slowly opened the dressing, a spurt of blood greeted us; it's making a small stream extending out almost two feet with each heartbeat. I used my left thumb, with light pressure, to stop the flow of blood enabling me to remove the bandage.

Sergio had cut through and amputated the left index and middle finger at the midknuckle. The ring finger is partially severed at the first joint. It's hanging and attached by the smallest piece of skin.

This is a serious injury as it involves so much of the left hand.

Sergio grimaced through the initial assessment. I placed the partially severed ring finger back into its anatomical position and wrapped it with moistened dressings, and Brad splinted the lower arm with a cardboard splint.

"Well, Sergio, we're going to take you to the hospital and have them help you, sound like a plan to you?" I said.

"Uh-huh," he said and trailed off.

The nurse handed me a brown paper bag with, "SERGIO-FINGERS" printed in red letters across the front of it.

I opened it and they have the two severed fingers wrapped in gauze in a baggie and then another larger baggie with ice chips surrounding it.

"Good job, and the labeling too," I said.

"Thanks, and thanks for being here," she said while wiping her brow with the back of her right hand.

Steve came over and said both students who passed out were feeling better.

"We'll hang out here until their parents arrive if you guys want to head out," he said.

"That sounds good, we should kind of get moving that way," I said.

I contacted dispatch on the portable radio and cancelled Eric's medic unit.

We have Sergio loaded onto the stretcher and headed to RGH.

"Sergio, do you need anything for the pain?" I asked.

"Uh…I think so, it's pretty bad," he said softly.

"Okay, well I'm going to start an IV in your right hand, do you understand me?" I asked.

"Is it going to hurt?" he asked.

I said, "Well, maybe just for a second, but I think you'll be okay, I'll do it fast."

It was ironic to think: *Here's a kid that just cut his fingers off and wondering if the IV will hurt.*

Sergio was a trooper on the IV, a slight wince and it was in. Over the next few hours, he'd appreciate this was in. Pain medication for this injury would certainly be indicated and he would always need just a little bit more than was he getting.

I started the morphine and would have 10 mg in by the time we arrived RGH.

Brad was in the middle of everything: checking blood pressures, writing information down, and answering questions for Sergio. We're lucky to have him today.

We got Sergio to the ED and directed to suite 6, and his mother arrived just after we did.

Sergio went to the OR and underwent reattachment surgery for the severed fingers. The surgeons were optimistic about the prognosis.

Back at the station, Steve, Sam, and Dana described their successful hand off the lightheaded kids to their parents. Steve and Dana ended up having to write a report on each of their patients.

Anytime you have a patient encounter, and they decline transport a report has to be written. It will include everything that goes into a typical transport case and then additional documentation about the reason for no transport. In this case, since the patients were minors, the parents had to sign a form indicating they were aware of risks that could be involved with no transport. The risks would be minimal but documentation is documentation.

After lunch, I got to spend some time with Brad and Rocky going over equipment in the ambulance. When the volunteers came into ride, we wanted to make their experience as valuable as possible.

I highlighted our LifePak 12 and discussed scenarios such as a patient with chest pain and being able to look at a 12-lead EKG which cannot only show us the heart attack but also what part of the heart that's being affected. This is crucial information to relay to the hospital and getting the cardiac team alerted.

In midsentence, Sandy appeared at the backdoors of the medic unit.

"Hey, Sandy, what's up?" I said.

"Well, there's a pickup truck in the parking lot and a man honking his horn. You might want to go see if he needs help," she said.

"Sure, we'll go check it out," I said.

Steve, Sam, and Dana also followed as we went through the pedestrian door to the public parking lot.

As we approached the vehicle, an elderly man in the driver's seat is waving from his open window. We notice blood streaming from along the bottom of the driver's door that created quite the puddle on the ground.

"Hi there, can we help you?" I asked.

"I cut myself with the chainsaw," he said with a pursed lip and tilt of the head.

I turned to Rocky and said, "Bring the ambulance around here, and we might want to expedite that."

"Roger that," he said.

Steve got on his portable radio and called dispatch.

"Could you place Medic 42 and Rescue 41 out of service for a drive up here at Station 4, we have an injured person and will advise further."

Dispatch confirmed the request.

"Okay, where did it get you?" I asked.

"My leg, it's pretty bad too," he said looking down at his leg.

As I peek in through the open window, there's blood everywhere. On the seat, the steering wheel, the dash, and a deep pool on the floor—everywhere.

Steve opened the driver's door slowly and blood flowed onto the ground like a flood gate had been opened. The man has a large towel wrapped from just above his right knee almost to the right hip and it's soaked in blood. It looks like he was butchered.

I'm not moving the towel until Rocky brings the medic unit around and we have equipment.

His radial pulse is faint at 130 beats. His skin is clammy and pale, he's breathing fast, and he's in shock. From the amount of blood visible, it's a miracle he has any left in his body.

Sam and Brad have large trauma dressings ready. I decided it might be better if we get him out the vehicle onto the gurney where we have more room to work.

"What is your name, sir?" I asked.

"Glen," he said.

"Okay, Glen, we're going to lift you out of there and set you on our gurney, you ready?" I said.

"Let's just go," he said.

There's even more blood that has become thick coagulated clumps on the seat. We now have him on the gurney and quickly into the back of the medic unit.

Steve is cutting clothing, and we're ready to examine the wound. Dana has an oxygen mask over Glen's mouth and nose, and Rocky is setting up an IV bag.

The wound is massive. It starts from just above the right knee and curves around toward the right hip. Its several inches wide with significant muscle and tissue damage and what looks like arterial flow from the midthigh.

This is a major injury and can rapidly become life threatening.

Sam and Brad placed their large trauma dressings over the gaping and actively flowing areas.

Brad placed two additional dressings over those while wrapping them around the leg and pulling the gaping tissues back together. He secured all the dressings with tightly wrapped stretch gauze.

"You got that pretty tight there my friend," Glen said.

"Well you have a pretty big opening there, Glen," Brad said with a reassuring smile.

I hear Rocky's door close, and we feel the rig accelerate, we're headed to a much-anticipated greeting at RGH.

I put the rubber tourniquet on Glen's left arm. It took a few minutes for a vein to appear and then placed a 16 gauge in it. The IV bag is hooked up and flowing.

Glen told us he was cutting large branches above his head when the saw unexpectedly bucked downward and into his right leg. He walked for several minutes to his truck and drove to the station. All this happened twenty minutes before he arrived at our station.

Glen is eighty-two years old.

Dana has the LifePak 12 hooked up and is calling numbers.

"Heart rate at 134, blood pressure 60/36, and SpO2 isn't reading," she said.

These are critical vitals.

We arrived at RGH where the trauma team took over. Glen quickly went to the OR, and after two hours, he was admitted to the trauma ICU.

We would hear later he was discharged to an extended care facility after five days and expected a complete recovery.

At the end of the day, Brad thanked us for the experience.

"You can't say we didn't get our share of trauma calls today," I said.

"No, I think I've seen enough blood and excitement for a couple shifts," he conceded.

Brad was about to leave the station when the tones resonated throughout the building.

"Rescue 41, Medic 42, respond code three for a seventy-one-year-old male with chest pain, #8 Meadow Lane, time out 1630 hours."

Rocky and I walked into the truck bay and looked back at Brad.

"Might as well come on one more call, sounds like we may get to use the LifePak 12," I said.

Brad dropped his bag and hopped in the side door of the ambulance.

With the afternoon traffic starting to get heavy, it would take five minutes to arrive. Steve and crew were following us in Rescue 41.

As we turned onto Meadow Lane, a female is waving to us from halfway down the block.

Pulling in front of the residence we see a large sign on the front door: Oxygen in Use—No Smoking.

This gave us information about the patient or someone in the house having medical issues serious enough to require supplemental oxygen.

As we got to the front door, the lady smiled nervously and said, "It's my husband, he's having chest pain and I'm worried about him."

"Okay, we'll check him out and see what's going on," I said.

We followed her to the kitchen where the patient was sitting.

He has his arms on the dining table with considerable focus on getting a breath. His color is ashen and he's anxious. He's wearing his nasal cannula oxygen tubing with the prongs that fit into his nose, and we hear hissing indicating its delivering oxygen.

"He has COPD," his wife said.

COPD is chronic obstructive pulmonary disease. It's usually emphysema but can also include chronic bronchitis. Emphysema is a progressive disease where the air sacs in the lungs, the alveoli, become damaged and unable to carry out oxygen intake or completely get rid of carbon dioxide. It's a vicious cycle and eventually the patient requires additional oxygen twenty-four hours a day.

He's in a classic position we see with COPD. The arms outstretched resting on the table allows the chest to expand easier and more air exchange to take place. This is also known as the tripod position.

"Hello, my name is Mark, I'm a paramedic, and can you tell me your name, sir?" I asked.

"Pete," he said.

"What's going on today?" I asked.

"I'm having some pain, here," he said and then put the palm of his hand to his chest and covers a large area of it.

"When did this start, Pete?" I asked.

"A couple hours ago, I took some nitros and they aren't helping," he said while obviously struggling and becoming more short of breath.

"Well, we're going to help you, I want to get you hooked up to our EKG and look at your heart," I said.

Dana and Brad were getting the LifePak 12 ready when Pete suddenly began to stand up.

This brought immediate concern from all us as we tried to stop his effort.

"Pete, I need you to stay still for a couple minutes," Dana explained.

"I have to go to the toilet," Pete said while continuing the effort and not slowing down.

"Pete, if you could hold off on that, we really need to see what's going on with your chest," I said.

It's not uncommon for patients with chest pain and even ongoing heart attacks to have the feeling or sensation they need to go the toilet. This can be disastrous as they can pass out while sitting on the commode or even have cardiac arrest.

With a burst of energy and almost combative charge, he stood up and walked into the hallway.

His wife yelled out, "Pete, let them check you please," she pleaded.

And in the next second, he was in the bathroom with the door closed and lock pressed.

We all looked at each and walked toward the bathroom door.

I got next to the door and spoke, "Pete, I understand you need to go, but it's really important we make sure you're going to be okay…can you hear me?" I said.

"Pete?" I called again, silence.

There's no response.

The next sound we heard elevated this situation to the worst-case scenario. Pete collapsed onto the floor, and we could hear agonal gasps. This means he may have coded and went into cardiac arrest.

A quick twist of the door handle, locked.

I looked at his wife and said, "Do you have a key or way to get in here?"

"No, he's never done this before," she said.

Steve dropped down to a knee in front of the door with his trusty all-purpose utility knife. He got it between the door and the frame, and with a quick shudder, the door sprung open.

Pete had collapsed in a position that meant we couldn't fully open the door. Steve and Brad squeezed through the opening, and lifted Pete as Dana opened the door. They carried Pete to the kitchen floor where Sam started compressions.

During the first few compressions, the familiar sound of cartilage separating between the ribs echoed through the kitchen. It's always an unsettling sound.

Steve cut Pete's shirt off, and Brad placed the rectangular combo pads on the chest and plugged the cable into the LifePak 12.

Rocky has the kit open, setting up an IV, and getting cardiac drugs prepared. Dana has the bag valve mask over Pete's face delivering breaths after Sam completes every thirty compressions.

"Sam, after this set of compressions, I want you and Brad to switch roles. Then we'll see what we got on the monitor," I said.

Sam nodded while focusing on the compressions, arms locked, and her shoulders squared over the top of Pete's sternum, all with perfect form.

"Okay, stop, Sam, V-fib…let's shock at 200…clear," as the shock was given, Pete arched at the energy.

Brad resumed compressions.

I placed a rubber tourniquet over Pete's upper left arm. He has a good vein in the midarm and I put a 14 gauge into it. Rocky handed me epinephrine, which I will give through the IV line after the next shock if we need it.

"All right, we're about ready to check the rhythm again. Steve, you take over for Brad after this check," I said.

"Roger that," Steve acknowledged.

"Okay, let's switch. V-fib…lets shock at 300 this time… clear," and the shock is delivered.

Time to get him intubated.

Dana is moving to the side as I'm above Pete's head. With the laryngoscope in my left hand, I slowly get the blade into his mouth when his top dentures come loose and become wedged toward the back of his throat.

I'm having difficulty getting a grip on them and can't immediately hook them with the blade. I seem to be stuck and by the smallest obstacle.

Dana reaches over with her small little fingers and with a quick pinch they're out.

Now, the second attempt without the obstruction and a great view of the vocal cords, the endotracheal tube is securely in place.

Dana is at the top of Pete's head with the bag valve attached to the tube and controlling the ventilations.

"Brad, I am going to have you back doing compressions after this check," I said.

"Roger that," Brad replied causing Steve to look at him and then me with a scrunched brow.

"Okay, let's switch and check this rhythm. Still V-fib...lets shock at 360...clear," and the shock is delivered.

I suddenly see Pete moving and grimacing at the compressions.

"Can you feel a pulse, Dana? I asked.

"Oh yeah, a good strong one," she said with two fingers on Pete's left carotid, pen in hand getting ready to place the 'X.'

"Very good, let's check a blood pressure, get ready to start moving to the ambulance," I said.

"Heart rate 104, blood pressure 80/62, and SpO2 84%," Brad called out.

These are very good numbers compared to where were a few minutes ago. They should improve as the heart continues to beat.

I have a few seconds to talk to his wife as the crew is carefully transferring Pete to the ambulance.

"We have his heart started again, I don't want to give you any false hopes, he's still very critical," I explained.

"I understand," she said.

"He's been fighting this for the last two years, thank you all for everything, I know you all are working very hard for him," she said with the warmest smile.

"You're welcome. We'll be going to Regional. Do you have a way to get there?" I asked.

"I called my daughter. She'll be here any second now," she said.

Pete continued to improve during the transport. His 12-lead EKG showed an ongoing injury pattern to the lower portion of his heart. We radioed this information ahead to the awaiting cardiac team.

"Heart rate 96, blood pressure 106/74, and SpO2 at 90%," Brad announced.

"That sounds great, Brad," I said.

"Thanks for staying and helping us, you do good work," I added.

Brad nodded and offered a humbled smile.

We got to RGH and handed Pete off to the awaiting cardiac team. He was quickly evaluated and then to the cath lab. He would have two stents placed and admitted to the CCU.

Back at the station, Brad thanked all us for having patience and letting him be part of the crew. We all agreed he could come back anytime. He got some invaluable experience today and made a difference in people's lives, that's why we're here.

The next shift, we came on duty and after getting the truck checks completed, Sam asked if I heard any updates on Pete. I told her I hadn't but we'd check if we made it to the hospital today.

Later that morning, we'd finished a short training session and were still in the training room when Sandy came in. "You guys have a visitor, a lady says you helped her husband, Pete, and she'd like to meet with all you," she said.

I walked with Sandy to the front office to escort Pete's wife back to the training room.

As I walked into the front office area, I suddenly felt as if this wasn't what we thought it might be.

"Hello, Mark," she said with a heavy voice and warm smile.

"It's very nice to see you, is Pete okay?" I asked.

She took moment to collect her next thought and after a slow cleansing breath said, "Pete died last night. My daughter and I were with him and it was very peaceful."

I stared at her, and walked over and we hugged for several seconds.

"I want to thank you all very much for everything you did. I saw how hard you all worked and were so careful with him. He was very sick and didn't have too many good days. I know he's okay now," she said.

"It means a lot for you to come here and tell us, I'm very sorry for your loss," I said.

"Will you please talk to your friends and tell them how much my daughter and I appreciate what they did?" she asked with sincerity.

"I will, and we'll keep you in our thoughts and please, let us know if we can do anything," I said.

After another hug and smile, she walked out the door and got into her daughter's car.

Sandy looked at me with her head tilted and quickly looked away as if she had something pressing to do at her desk. Her cheek glistened with a single tear.

I walked back to the training room, as soon as I walked in everyone knew what the visit was about. We talked about it as a crew and thought about Pete several times throughout the day.

Joe has reminded us over the years, "Every call is a chance to make a difference in someone's life."

7

BON VOYAGE

Rocky and Rachel were given a two-week cruise, all expenses paid including airfare by a generous family member. After arranging time off, they were fortunate to have Ariel volunteer to house sit and take care of Hank, Abby, and Kelsey.

Sam is stepping up to be my partner on Medic 42 and excited about the change of pace from the rescue.

Nick Caffrey is one of our star EMT volunteers and will cover Sam's position on the rescue. He has been with Station 4 the last two years and a veteran EMT. Nick has a strong interest in becoming more involved with the department, and this is a great opportunity for him.

Two things we never seem to get enough of, training and paperwork. As prehospital care providers, we have to recertify at our respective certification levels, paramedic, EMT, every two years. This process also involves having a number of continuing educational hours.

We've covered our required topics for the month and now have flexibility in our topics.

With Nick being part of the team, I wanted him to become more familiar with the kits we use on scene.

Our main kit can be intimidating as it's packed with literally everything we could need on a scene until we can get the patient into the medic unit.

I labeled a blank sheet of paper with the alphabet down the left side and called the crews into the training room.

"Okay, we all have a good working knowledge of the main kit, I want you list everything that's in the kit next to the letter, and you have fifteen minutes," I explained.

"I don't understand," Sam said looking at me like a deer facing headlights.

"Like *blood pressure cuff* would go under the 'B', *epinephrine* would go under the 'E'," I said.

"Oh, I get it, well that's pretty simple," she said and started writing.

After fifteen minutes, we compared papers. It was comical on some of the letters. Nick was naming everything he had under the 'N' and the first thing he said was, "Narcan."

Sam pounded the desk and covered her eyes, "Oh man, how could I forget that one," she laughed.

It was a great exercise and the tones broke the mood.

"Rescue 41, Medic 42, respond code three for an unresponsive fourteen-year-old female, 1714 Rock Point Road, time out 0855 hours."

Both units quickly went en route. Today's a school day, someone must be pretty sick to call an ambulance to get out of going to school.

Sam had us on scene in less than four minutes and parked behind a patrol car. Walking up to the front door, a well-dressed female met us with a worried and frantic expression.

"Please, it's my daughter, she's locked in her room," she explained.

Just then the police officer appeared from a short stairway and after exchanging nods with us, said, "I'm not sure what we have here, I knocked on the door and didn't get any response."

"Can you tell us more about why you think she may be in trouble?" I asked the mother.

"We had a pretty bad fight at six this morning about her schoolwork and a boy she's seeing. She stormed off to her room and locked the door. She hasn't come out since and this is way beyond her normal behavior," she explained.

"Has she ever tried to hurt herself?" I asked with as much sensitivity as possible.

"Well no, I mean she makes threats when she gets upset, everyone does, why are you asking?" she asked with an obvious increasing anxiety level.

"Well, I think we need to get into the room, we may have to force the door if that's okay?" I asked.

"Do whatever you need to," she said while starting to show an uncomfortable concern.

"What's her name?" I asked.

"Ginny, she's fourteen," her mother said.

We walked down the short flight of stairs and stood in front of Ginny's door. The officer stood next to the door and pounded several times announcing we were going to force if she didn't open it.

There was no response. He tried the door handle again before putting a quick forceful shoulder to it which cracked the frame and sprung the door open.

Ginny is lying in bed on her left side. There's a small pile of vomit next to her face. Her face is ashen gray and her breathing is rapid and deep.

She's wearing black stretch pants to midshin, no shoes or socks, a pink tank top, and clutching a photo of a young male in her left hand.

There's a pill bottle on the nightstand with the top off and a large, nearly empty glass of water next to it.

She doesn't respond to us being in the room.

I picked up the bottle, and as I read the label, my heart sank. It's Elavil, a powerful antidepressant and deadly to overdose on. It's part of a class of drugs known as tricyclic antidepressants or TCAs.

The label has a pill count of thirty and filled two days ago. It's empty.

"That's my husband's medication, where did she get that?" Her mother shouted.

At this point, it isn't important where she got it; we need to get moving if we're going to have any chance of saving Ginny.

Dana has the LifePak 12 hooked up.

"Heart rate 136, blood pressure 70/44, SpO2 88%," she said.

This is getting worse by the second. The high heart rate and pattern of the EKG indicate Ginny probably took all the pills and they've been in her system for a while.

Sam and Steve were bringing the gurney into the house.

"Have them keep it upstairs. We'll carry her up to them," I said to Dana as she quickly exited the room.

Nick and I easily carried Ginny up the stairs to the gurney. Dana positioned Ginny's head to where her breathing wasn't obstructed, and we're ready to move to the ambulance.

I had a few seconds to speak to her mother.

"I want to be honest with you, this is an extremely dangerous drug she's taken, and we need to get her to the hospital, quickly. The officer can help you but we have to leave now," I said.

"Is she going to be okay?" she asked with an innate fear in her voice.

"We're doing everything we can right now, we need to get her to the hospital," I repeated trying to offer reassurance yet not give false hopes.

We've had people over the years overdose on Elavil and the outcomes are not good. There's no antidote for an overdose of Elavil once it's in the system.

In the ambulance, I quickly got an IV started on Ginny's left arm. I drew up the drugs for the RSI procedure, and as they went in, Ginny responded quickly and ready for the intubation. She's an easy intubation and Dana is now in charge of ventilating her.

Her vital signs are getting worse.

"Heart rate 154, blood pressure 60/24, SpO2 isn't reading," Nick called out.

We're all very aware of how sick Ginny is and where this is heading.

If you want to see something impressive, watch a medic crew working in the back of a mobile intensive care unit not accepting of an almost certain outcome.

We arrived at RGH and the ED staff flew into action continuing this aggressive direction as Ginny deteriorated quickly.

Twenty-two minutes after we arrived, she went into cardiac arrest.

Dr. Stein continued the resuscitation for seventy-four agonizing minutes before making the toughest decision to stop the efforts.

Ginny was pronounced dead at 1059 hours.

The numbness that follows this call will last a few days, and probably never completely goes away.

The next shift, Sam and I spent a lot of time during the morning vehicle inspection talking in the back of the ambulance. Before long, Dana, Nick, and Steve were also huddled in the back with us.

This turned into an incredibly therapeutic healing session after the last several shifts of very difficult calls.

Steve was telling us stories about guys in his military unit that had us crying with laughter, and after almost three hours, we suddenly realized how long we'd been in the back of the ambulance.

Not sure how we did it, but we felt recharged and like we'd be okay for the next round.

Nick made us lunch with grilled cheese sandwiches and tomato soup, and Sam showed everyone the correct ratios for dipping bread and soup. This would be one of the lighter moments around the station, certainly not reflective of the highly trained and professional rescuers that show up on a scene.

We finished lunch and had a relaxing afternoon with no calls. It couldn't last forever before the tones reverberated through the station, back to reality.

"Rescue 41, Medic 42, respond code three for an unconscious male, in a vehicle, 3400 block of Orlando Street, time out 1602 hours.

The bay doors for Rescue 41 were rolling up as Sam activated the siren, hit the overhead lights and headed that way. Orlando Street would be a four-minute response.

For at least a half mile up the road, I can see brake lights and cars pulling to the right and stopping.

"Wow, Rocky doesn't have it that lucky, what's your secret?" I asked.

"They've probably seen me at the gun range," Sam said and looked at me from the corners of her eyes grinning.

We hear police traffic on the scanner requesting EMS to expedite as the patient is bleeding heavily.

Turning onto Orlando Street, we see two patrol cars parked next to a vehicle that's nose first into a utility pole. The vehicle looks as if it stopped against the pole versus crashing into it. There's no damage to the car or the pole.

Walking up to the vehicle, we notice a large combat-type knife lying on the roof of the car with blood stained over the handle and length of the blade.

The patient is sitting in the driver's seat with his head tilted back and not moving. He looks lifeless with his eyes nearly closed, mouth half open and deathlike color.

One of the officers is leaning in through the driver's door holding a large blood-soaked dressing to the patient's left arm. The other officer has the passenger door open and holding a large blood-soaked dressing to the patient's right arm.

The officer at the driver's door nods to me and says, "I think this might be a first."

As I get a better view of the patient, there's a considerable amount of blood in his lap and coagulated clumps on the driver's seat. Both arms have at least twenty separate slicing-type wounds to the bone. There's an empty fifth of whiskey on the floor next to the brake pedal along with several empty bottles of aspirin.

Nick and Dana have large trauma dressings and have taken over for the officers.

The patient is ghostly pale with beads of sweat across his forehead and breathing is rapid. He's unresponsive to voice or taps to the shoulder. He doesn't have a radial pulse indicating his blood pressure is critically low.

There's a heavy alcohol eminence throughout the car.

The patient looks to be in his late twenties. There's no note of intent for this seemingly obvious yet still suspicious presentation, or wallet or any indication of who he is.

The officer later informed me the car is registered to a female.

Steve has the gurney next to the car. Sam is getting equipment setup in the ambulance.

Nick and Dana have the bleeding controlled, and we're ready to move him to the gurney.

Dana's in the passenger side and brought his legs up onto the seat. Steve and Nick are able to pull him straight out onto the stretcher.

I happen to notice he's making subtle motions as if he's about to vomit.

We moved the gurney a few feet away from the car and prepared to roll him on his side when he suddenly begins vomiting in quick successions. It's spraying out three to four feet and splashing wildly all over the road.

This is a volatile mixture of stomach contents; alcohol and what looked like a hundred pill fragments followed by the overpowering aroma.

He's now gasping for breaths intermixed with gurgling. Sam brought the portable suction unit and is doing a good job managing the secretions. He's starting to become blue about the face and lips which is raising red flags.

The officers are standing several feet away watching in almost disbelief.

This is a worst-case scenario of an unsecured airway spiraling out of control.

We moved to the back of the ambulance between vomiting episodes. Dana has an oxygen mask next to his face. Sam is working hard with the suction to clear the remaining fluid and chunks.

With the lacerations to his arms, I don't have any viable IV sites. He has a very large external jugular vein along the right side of his neck. This has to be the IV site. With the patient on his left side, the neck vein is easy to see and I put a 14 gauge into it.

I made a difficult decision to intubate him by using the RSI drugs. We're eight minutes from RGH, and I don't believe we can keep him from aspirating during that time with the unsecured airway.

Additionally, his poor color is indicative of hypoxia (lack of oxygen) which has him at significant risk for catastrophic brain or cardiac injury.

I do have one advantage on my side; anatomically, he doesn't have any obvious indications of a difficult intubation.

With the RSI drugs drawn up, Nick and Dana are in positions to provide ventilations with the bag valve mask if needed. Sam's in position with the suction wand, and Steve's ready to push the medications.

Within seconds, the patient has stopped breathing. Nick is holding gentle pressure over the lower part of the throat that will help in preventing passive vomiting. This is a controversial procedure, and critics go both ways on the efficacy of it.

As I slide the blade down the throat, Sam is providing suction to remove small food chunks that are obscuring my field of vision surrounding the vocal cords. She has perfected this assist, and I wouldn't be able to complete the procedure without her assistance.

I withdrew the laryngoscope blade after watching the tube go through the vocal cord opening and into the trachea. We're all breathing a sigh with the airway being secured.

Nick is now sitting in the jump seat, ventilating with the bag valve, staring intently ensuring each breath goes in.

During the reassessment, the lacerated arms have stopped bleeding and there are no other injuries I can find.

We brought the five empty pill bottles of aspirin along with the empty whiskey bottle. The officers took control of the knife.

"Heart rate 118, blood pressure 66/54, SpO2 90%, and blood sugar is 102," Dana called out.

"Roger that, thanks, Dana," I said.

Considering the amount of blood loss, the vital signs could be worse. He's still critical with the aspirin in his system. Even though he had several episodes of vomiting, there's no way to tell how much is still in there or already absorbed.

As we arrived at RGH, we had plenty of help getting him into suite 12. The gastric lavage was set up quickly. This would be a procedure to remove stomach contents quickly.

It wasn't long before they have more pill fragments coming up through the lavage tube. This was eventually used to administer activated charcoal in an attempt to have whatever was left in the stomach pass through the digestive system without being absorbed.

After having tendons in both arms repaired in the OR, he's admitted to the ICU. The next twenty-four hours will determine whether he survives this incident or succumbs to it. His blood alcohol level on admission is .32.

The patient is thirty years old. He has a history of depression and previous suicide attempts. They believe this attempt was precipitated by a recent breakup with his girlfriend of two years.

Driving back to the station looked like rush hour and it's almost 2000 hours. Most of the drivers and passengers are responsible and having a good time which doesn't involve meeting law enforcement or EMS. Unfortunately, some will fit into that category, and for a few, it could be their final night.

Sam got the ambulance restocked in anticipation of a busy night and taking advantage of the lull.

We're relaxed in the day room, chairs reclined and even a few snores to be heard.

Dana has the remote control, slowly going through the lineup of channels for the third time.

This hypnotic trance she seems entwined in was suddenly broken by tones that provided a shot of adrenalin, snapping everyone back to reality and heading to the bays.

"Rescue 41, Medic 42, respond code three to the area of Williams Road and Sunset View for a reported motor vehicle crash, time out 2354 hours."

As we left the station, traffic seems to have gotten worse, or at least no better.

"Geez people, go home, go to bed," Sam exclaimed.

Sounded like a good advice to me.

After responding for several minutes, we receive an update from dispatch.

"Rescue 41, Medic 42, deputies are on scene and advising one patient, DOA."

Steve and I both received the update and advised our (estimated time of arrival) ETA would be less than two minutes. It sounded like one of the drivers from tonight wouldn't be going home.

We arrived on scene and saw the rear end of a pickup truck off the road and crashed head on into a large tree. There are two cars parked ahead of the crash, the drivers are standing next to each other. By the looks on their faces, they must have been first on scene and made the 9-1-1 call.

The pickup truck driver is a young male. His color is pale and lifeless. He's heavily pinned in the crushed interior of the cab. From what we can see, he has massive chest and open head injuries that are very graphic. He's not wearing a seat belt and a strong alcohol aroma is coming from the cab.

He has no carotid pulse and isn't making any attempt to breathe; based on the obvious injuries, we're not going to attempt resuscitation.

The injuries associated with this type of collision include fatal brain trauma, ruptured aortas, cervical neck fractures, and ruptured spleens and livers. Death can be almost instantaneous. The extrication alone could take fifteen minutes or longer depending on the degree of entrapment once we started tearing the vehicle apart.

As we're getting ready to climb the shallow embankment to the road, Sam suddenly freezes in step and holds her right clenched fist up. We instinctively stop and look at her with puzzled stares.

Nick now has the same look as Sam and starts to walk back down the embankment beyond the truck into a grouping of small trees.

We have flashlights trying to pierce the inky black of the night looking for the origin of what sounded like a moans.

After a few seconds, Nick calls out, "Over here guys, we have another patient."

Deputies would later find out through investigation the pickup's driver left a party to go purchase more alcohol. He left with another male who was standing in the truck's open bed, over the cab with arms outstretched like he was flying. When they didn't return, everyone assumed they'd gone to another party.

He is our patient, found nearly twenty-five feet from the crash. He's lying face up and choking on blood in between forced moans. He's unresponsive to our shouts or taps to the shoulders.

His most graphic presentation is the small tree branch impaled into his right lower abdomen. It's approximately four inches long and buried deep into the stomach. We won't remove it in this setting.

His right leg is bent at the midthigh and tucked beneath him. He's breathing rapidly at over forty times a minute and frequently interrupted by the choking. His lungs sound clear and equal. He has no radial pulse so we know his blood pressure is less than 80, his carotid pulse is 130 beats per minute, and there's a heavy alcohol aroma coming from his breath.

Nick has taken control of the patient's head with his hands along the ears. Sam headed back to the ambulance for the gurney and long spine board and more equipment.

Dana is using the suction unit to clear blood that's collecting in his mouth.

We need to get him packaged and into the back of the ambulance in order to secure the airway.

Steve has all the clothing cut away. I'm going to take control of the right leg as we roll him onto his left side. Sam has the long spine board ready and next to him.

During the move, we have a chance to inspect the back. The branch has not gone all the way through the abdomen. Bringing the right leg back to the anatomical position is very graphic with the unmistakable sounds of the bone ends grinding together.

The right femur fracture is secured under the straps from the long spine board.

With the help of the deputies, we're able to carry him on the spine board through the unstable ground and get him to the gurney and into the back of the ambulance.

We've been on scene for thirteen minutes.

Dana has an oxygen mask over his mouth and nose. She's also suctioning as needed with the bleeding. Nick has the LifePak 12 hooked up and the numbers are not encouraging.

"Heart rate 140, blood pressure 66/40, SpO2 at 80%," he called out.

"Roger that," I said with full focus and awareness of where this is heading.

After applying the rubber tourniquet to the left arm, I found a good vein in the midarm and put a 14 gauge into it.

We can now prepare the RSI drugs and get the airway secured.

Dana yelled out, "I think he just coded."

Looking over at the monitor shows a bizarre-looking rhythm, and no corresponding pulse. It's an agonal or dying rhythm, a worst-case scenario.

One of the main reasons for this activity is the body running out of blood. The heart wants to beat, but there isn't any fluid to pump.

It's a frightful and difficult presentation to fix outside the OR and rarely a successful resuscitation.

Dana began compressions. I'm at the patient's head and preparing to intubate. We won't need the RSI procedure now.

As I introduce the laryngoscope, I'm immediately presented with copious amounts of blood and pieces of tongue. Nick is focusing with the suctioning and it is difficult.

After several seconds, I can see the vocal cords and see the tube pass through them.

Nick is now ventilating as Dana is compressing the chest. It's a dangerous resuscitation in a moving ambulance.

I have the IV bag flowing wide open and desperately searching for a second site. I found a smaller vein in the right lower arm and put a 16 gauge into it.

The second IV bag is flowing wide open.

We arrived at RGH to an awaiting trauma team that would continue the resuscitation effort for another thirty-two minutes before exhausting the chances of reversing the massive insult from the crash.

Our patient's name was Arlen. He was twenty-two years old and lost his life not only recklessly but also senselessly. Did he consider this when he chose to ride atop the cab of the truck?

As is often the case in EMS, we have more questions than we have answers for, tonight we added some to that list.

8

MENTAL HEALTH CHECK

WHEN YOU COME through those doors in the morning, you never know what kind of calls the shift will bring. Some days it's all medical, and some days all trauma, and some days it's all the above. Last shift, Sam and I had four diabetics, all unconscious with nearly the same low blood sugar readings, coincidence?

We're getting close to a full moon and as anyone in EMS will tell you, beware. The cynics will dismiss it as chance but every dispatcher, medic, police officer, or ED nurse with tenure will testify differently.

Today will begin right out of the chute, no time to get the rigs checked before the tones have us headed out.

"Rescue 41, Medic 42, respond code three for a car versus pedestrian, 801 Colorado Street, police on scene, time out 0808."

Traffic is heavy this morning but we should be there in less than four minutes.

As we're arriving, we count three patrol cars with one of them blocking a lane of travel.

Over on the sidewalk, the officers are involved in a fierce and violent struggle with a person on the ground. One of them has the guy by the legs and the other two are trying to control his arms and the suspect doesn't seem fazed by any of it.

This will turn out to be our patient.

We would learn the police have been looking for this man for the last half hour. Several calls were made to 9-1-1 about a man acting strangely, barking at traffic, and crawling around on his hands and knees in the road.

He was finally struck by a car as he attempted to run alongside it while barking and trying to bite the side mirror.

When police arrived, he growled ferociously, bared teeth and started fighting with them.

The patient's name is Romeo. He's thirty-two years old and a local transient. He has a schizophrenic history, and as long as he's on his medication, he's quite harmless. Today, something upset that balance.

We expeditiously make our way to the scuffle as it's ending with the patient being cuffed.

Steve is maintaining Romeo's head and neck in line in case of a cervical spine injury as Nick is getting the cervical collar around his neck.

Sam has the long spine board, and we're able to get Romeo secured and strapped.

Dana is cutting clothing as I assess what injuries he may have sustained from being struck by the vehicle. He has abrasions to the chest, abdomen, and palms of the hand, that's all I can find.

His color is good, radial pulse is elevated at 120 but that can be secondary to the agitation. He hasn't said anything indicating he's aware of what's going on and doesn't respond to questions.

When a person is having pain from an external injury, it's obvious and treatment can be tangible as well as measureable.

When the pain is mental, it's difficult to offer the same definitive treatment path. It has to be agonizing, locked in a silent world that has you out of control mentally and emotionally.

As a crew, we understand this and do not judge the patient's actions, they're merely a reflection of this loss of rationality which takes a person to the edge of whatever the mind can summon.

It can be ostracized with unintentional ignorance as people fear what they cannot understand or see.

I placed an IV into the back of Romeo's right hand. This would allow me to administer medication to provide some respite from this nightmarish siege he's under.

His blood sugar level is 94.

EKG and blood pressure both look good. Romeo is fortunate he did not sustain serious injury or worse while experiencing this psychotic episode.

He spent several hours in the ED without visitors, family, or friends. His injuries were minor. He's admitted to the psychiatric floor with the goal of getting his medication level back to a therapeutic range.

Back at the station, we finished the daily vehicle checks. Our training room is just outside the large day room. We gathered in the day room in anticipation of our daily training when Sandy appeared with several elderly citizens walking behind her with attentive and curious looks.

"Here are our star medics and rescue crews," Sandy said with enthusiasm.

"These folks are from the community center and visiting the local businesses this morning," she explained.

"It's very nice to see you all and welcome to Station 4," I said.

"We appreciate you guys and what you do for our community," the gentleman in the front said.

"Well, that means a lot, and we appreciate the recognition, we take great pride in what we do," I said.

"Were getting ready to conduct a—" and this statement was interrupted.

The tones echoing through the station had some of them looking at the ceiling and two of them covering their ears and crouching as if it were an air raid siren alert.

"It was very nice to talk to you, and we look forward to seeing you in the future, duty calls," I said with a smile and we headed for the bays.

"Rescue 41, Medic 42, respond code three for an unconscious twenty-eight-year-old female, 1212 Rose Place, time out 1140 hours."

We've had calls in this area before, mostly for drug overdoses and assaults. The response would take only a few minutes.

Arriving in front of the residence, we're met by a man waving. I acknowledge him, and from his demeanor there doesn't seem to be any sense of urgency. As we're walking up to the front door, a police car is pulling up behind the rescue unit.

"Did you call us?" I asked.

"Yeah, it's my old lady, she won't wake up," he said.

The man is rail thin, no shirt, barefoot, and wearing only jeans with holes through the knees. His hair is greasy and uncombed. There are tattoos across his chest and neck that don't seem to make any sense, and he's hyperactive to the point of being unable to remain still for more than a couple seconds.

"Okay let's go check her out," I suggested.

Upon entering the house we have to negotiate our way through a maze of trash bags, bicycle parts, tires, and everything else that might be in our way. One of the trash bags has rustling inside it which startled Dana as she adjusted her step to walk farther from it. The house reeks of cigarettes, eye burning cat urine, and rotting food—a volatile and depressing combination.

Walking down a short hallway we come to a bedroom on the right. The room is dark with a blanket hung over the window and no working light. There's a bed, small table, and piles of clothes littering the floor and more bags of trash.

The female patient is naked, lying on her stomach on the right half of the bed.

She has rapid snoring respirations over sixty a minute, her arms are at her side with palms extended and legs and feet have the same extension pattern.

This is posturing, a grave presentation and indication of a brain injury. Swelling in the brain can cause the abnormal extensions in the extremities.

She's unresponsive to voice or gentle shake to the upper back.

The male is claiming he went to wake her two hours ago, and she was sleeping heavy. He checked later and after seeing no change became concerned and called 9-1-1.

He denies any type of complaint prior to her going to sleep and eventually admits she uses methamphetamine but "not that much."

"Nick, you and Dana carry her into the living room, we'll get a place cleared to put her," I said.

"Roger that, let's go, Dana," he said.

The patient is also rail thin, and while Nick and Dana prepare to lift her, they find the bed heavily soaked in urine.

Steve guided them as they cautiously made their way to the front room.

Sam was setting equipment up while I found an area for us to work. The patient gave no response to being carried.

Sam placed an oxygen mask over her mouth and nose. The problem was found very quickly upon checking the pupils. Her right pupil is blown indicating some massive intracranial insult happening, probably bleeding. This would explain the extension and posturing of the extremities. A blown pupil is a pupil nearly totally dilated, large, compared to the opposite one. It's indicative of swelling in the brain and an ominous sign. You're not conscious with a blown pupil which is a slang term.

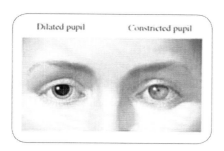

Dana is getting the LifePak 12 hooked up, and I'm placing an IV in the left arm. I'm going to RSI her and take control of her breathing which is still at near sixty a minute.

"Heart rate 46, blood pressure 180/120, SpO2 at 90%, and sugar is 88," Dana called out.

"Roger that," I said, "Let's go ahead and push the RSI drugs."

Within several seconds, she stopped breathing and was ready to be intubated. The procedure was quick and we're now ready to transport.

"Is she going to be okay?" the male asked.

"I don't know," I said, "She's very sick right now, and we need to get her to the hospital."

He paused as if to respond but instead turned toward the kitchen and grabbed a pack of cigarettes.

During the transport to RGH there are no changes. There's nothing more we can do other than get her to the hospital and the team.

As the results of the CT scan came back, it was as suspected, a massive bleed in the brain and will not be survivable.

She didn't make it out of the ED.

She coded thirty minutes after we arrived. They worked on her for another twenty-six minutes before pronouncing her dead. The boyfriend did not show up at the ED. She was alone in death.

She would have an autopsy and toxicological screen performed. It would show near fatal amounts of methamphetamine and heroin. Cause of death was listed as massive intracranial hemorrhage.

We got back to the station right at 1400 hours. The big choice now is to decide if we want a late lunch or early dinner. For some reason neither one sounded very appetizing.

As a county agency, we don't provide nonemergency services. In other words, we generally only respond to 9-1-1 generated calls. There are rare occasions when we can be taken out of service and cover that gap. Today we have one of those scenarios.

RGH has a limited amount of space in the psychiatric unit. They're currently at full capacity and cannot accept psychiatric patients for admission.

The tones started our adventure to the state mental hospital.

"Medic 42, respond code one to the ED at RGH for an emergency transfer, time out 1816 hours."

Sam and I headed that way with curiosity. This was a rare situation. We're updated no special equipment would be needed and the patient would be ready on our arrival.

We arrived at the ED and brought our gurney with us, it was strange walking through the door with an empty stretcher. We met with Brenda, the nursing supervisor, and got the full story.

"Hi guys, we have a forty-one-year-old gentleman who was brought in by police after having a severe psychiatric episode at a private residence. He fought with several officers before they had him under control. He's being admitted to the state mental hospital for a ninety-day evaluation for acute psychosis and homicidal ideations. He's heavily sedated after how violent he was and will remain restrained, they're expecting him," she explained.

The state mental hospital is about forty-five minutes from here. We've never been there but sounds like a pretty straightforward transfer. Besides, with him being sedated, he'll sleep the whole way and he's fully restrained.

We're headed to suite 6 and surprised to see the size of the patient. He's at least six-foot plus and well over two hundred pounds. He's asleep and doesn't stir as we enter the room. We begin the transfer from their stretcher to our gurney and it goes without incident.

After ensuring we have the paperwork and directions, we're ready to head out. Sam volunteered to ride in the back of the ambulance for the trip up there. This will give her some patient care time and she'll also complete the report.

After an uneventful trip, we're finally arriving on the grounds of the state hospital. The area is dimly lit and suddenly there are roads not reflected on the map Brenda supplied us with and we're "slightly" lost.

I asked Sam to navigate, she hopped up to the passenger seat, and both of us strained to find signs and landmarks that coincided with the map. In the pitch black of night with no street lights, it was becoming unsettling. After several minutes, we thought we might have it figured out.

That's when we both nearly had heart attacks.

"Where are we?" a strange voice called out.

Sam and I slowly looked over our shoulders to see the patient kneeling between us and peering out the front window acting like he's part of the crew. We slowly looked at each other with wide eyes and froze.

How did he get out of his restraints? Who knows…he did!

I noticed Sam had her hand on the door handle and was hoping she wouldn't jump out.

"Hey, how are you, we're almost there, you should probably go lay back down on the gurney," I said with my best happy voice.

"That's okay…I'm all right here…where we going?" he asked.

"What's your name?" he asked Sam a second later.

Sam is frozen, staring straight ahead. With the lighting from the instrument panel, I can see her firm grip on the door handle, knuckles becoming white.

About then we came around a corner and miraculously at the entrance to the admitting door. There are three big security guards standing there and one of them waved as we pulled up.

"Okay, we're here, you need to go sit on the gurney, hospital policy," I said.

"Okay, I'm hungry. Can I get something to eat in there?" he asked.

"Sure, just go lay back down," I said.

And with that he moved back.

I quickly set the ambulance in park and got out to talk to the guards. I think Sam's door actually opened a full second before I put the ambulance in park.

We opened the backdoors, and the patient is lying on the gurney with his arms behind his head. His eyes are dark and empty along with a surreal soul-piercing grin.

It was to say the least, unsettling.

Going into the facility we passed through several locked doors and finally made it out none the worse for the experience.

Sam drove us home and admitted she didn't want to do any more routine transfers.

I agreed.

We got back and Dana met us in the truck bay.

"How'd it go?" she asked.

Sam looked at her in passing and said, "Perfect, you got the next one, all yours," and walked into the day room.

Dana looked at me and said, "What happened, what's that supposed to mean?"

"Oh, the map wasn't exactly accurate," I said and then followed Sam into the day room.

Dana stood there scratching her head.

We caught up on paperwork and got several hours of sleep which was unusual for our station. Of course, the tones wouldn't let us have the entire night off.

"Rescue 41, Medic 42, respond and stage for a male subject threatening to shoot himself, law enforcement is responding, 18 Spruce Park Way, time out 0320 hours."

It would take several minutes to get to this address, and this will give law enforcement time to secure the scene.

We parked a block away from the scene and now sit and wait patiently.

We have (mobile data transmitters) MDTs in the ambulance and rescue. This allows us to receive updated information about the call which shows up on the screen.

This patient is thirty-six years old and has a schizophrenic history. A (mental health professional) MHP case worker contacted police after she learned the patient had gone off his medication, made suicidal threats, and literally destroyed his apartment.

A safety caution has been issued as the patient is violent, strong, and could be dangerous to responding personnel.

I got out of the ambulance and walked back to the rescue. I wanted to make sure Steve, Nick, and Dana had the information and we're all on the same page. As I was talking to them, we got an update from dispatch.

"Rescue 41, Medic 42, police requesting you respond into the scene, the patient has a gunshot wound to the chest."

Steve and I both received the update and drove around the block to the scene. There are two patrol cars across the street and two in front of the residence.

Walking into the house, there's a light blue haze of gun smoke along with the smell gunpowder in the air.

There are four officers actively fighting with the patient. He has jeans on and no shirt. The fight is ferocious as the officers are trying to get him restrained. Nick and Steve join in and between the six of them get the patient handcuffed with his hands behind him and laying on his right side.

The patient has a small single penetrating wound just below the left nipple with powder burns surrounding it and trickle of blood coming from it.

I listen to his chest with the stethoscope and can hear clear and equal lung sounds. There's no exit wound I can see.

The patient is calm, staring vacantly straight ahead, blinking, oblivious to all this.

His right radial pulse is 120 beats per minute.

He did just get done fighting so it could be high from adrenalin or worse, blood loss. His color is good, no signs of shock.

It's a confusing presentation.

In fact, he looks completely normal other than the hole in his chest and hands behind his back, handcuffed.

Sam has the long spine board and gurney ready. We'll need to put him in full spinal precautions as we don't know where the bullet ended up. If it's in the spine, it could still end up doing permanent damage.

With an officer on each extremity, the left cuff is removed, and he's secured on the spine board; each hand is cuffed to the board, at his side. He doesn't as much as move a muscle during this.

The patient will not answer questions and continues to stare blankly. With his current mental state, he's still very dangerous and unpredictable.

We also have to remember he's not acting with conscious reason. He's in an extremely delusional state.

As we're lifting the spine board to the gurney, he suddenly erupts and fighting against the cuffs and seatbelts. The display of strength is challenging the belts but holding him flat.

Dana and Nick are struggling to keep him from pulling his head up off the spine board.

As quickly as it begins he abruptly stops and relaxes.

We are headed to RGH and have one of the officers with us. If we need the cuffs off for any lifesaving issue, he's right there and the added safety factor doesn't hurt.

I need IV access and found a large vein in the right midarm. It went in without a flinch from the patient.

Dana has the LifePak 12 hooked up and is calling the current vital signs.

"Heart rate 104, blood pressure 160/100, and SpO2 99%," she said.

We arrived at RGH with a heavy security presence and quickly into suite 12. The patient was secured to the gurney with both soft restraints and leather restraints for the legs.

The initial chest x-ray shows the bullet just under the skin. It hit the fifth rib and ricochets two inches to the left and didn't penetrate the chest cavity.

The line it would have followed could have taken it through the heart and undoubtedly been fatal. He'll have the bullet removed in suite 12 under a local anesthetic.

The patient was admitted to the psychiatric unit and heavily sedated. He would make a full recovery and was remanded to the state mental hospital for a ninety-day evaluation.

9

BACK TO FULL STAFF

Rocky and Rachel finished their cruise. Today is his first shift back after two weeks off. Between being seasick and having the only weeks of the entire year with inclement weather, they had a great time.

"Did you guys do anything exciting without me?" Rocky asked.

"Oh, we had a few calls, nothing unusual," I said. "Nice to have you back though."

"We could get used to the cruises," Rocky mused.

"They have paramedics and EMTs, we'd fit right in," he added.

"Well, I guess we always have something to fall back on," I said.

Rocky was about to add more when the tones went off.

"Rescue 41, Medic 42, respond code three for an accidental ingestion, 24 Sun View Drive, time out 0818 hours."

As usual we're quick out of the large bay doors and Sun View Drive is a four-minute response. Traffic is heavy coming into town; heading out of town gives us the advantage. We have the ubiquitous stares as we race by motorists heading to their jobs and destinations, momentarily distracted while they wonder where we're going and what tragedy is unfolding at this hour of the day.

"Rescue 41, Medic 42, be advised your patient is a two-year-old male. He has ingested an unknown substance, caller is frantic. We are trying to get additional information."

Steve and I both acknowledged the update.

We're turning onto Sun View Drive, and see an elderly female standing in the doorway of a residence a few doors down, she's holding a child and waving as we pull in front of the home.

"I didn't know what to do. Dear God, this is bad, please tell me everything is going to be okay," she said as we walked up to the front door.

"Okay, my name is Mark, I'm a paramedic, and can you give us a little more information, what happened?" I asked as we made our way into the house.

The child looks okay from the initial appearance. He has good color, taking in the commotion, and looking around with curiosity at these strange people and grandma so worried; he does have what looks like flecks of mud around his mouth, nose, and on both hands.

The house is littered with toys scattered around the room in what otherwise looks like a very clean and well-maintained home. Two cats are sitting on the window ledge, watching as if they are amused by the distraction in their otherwise solitary lives.

She took a few deliberate breaths, closed her eyes in a forced relaxing state and then spoke.

"This is Skyler. He's my grandson. My daughter brought him here an hour ago, I was washing my hands and left him for just a few seconds," she explained.

"That's when he did it," she said, and then started crying.

This is painstakingly slow trying to figure out what we're dealing with here. We're standing in a "ready mode," waiting to spring into action and begin treatment when we finally get to the emergency.

"I found him at the litter box, he, he ate some of the, some of the, *pieces*," she said and then really broke down and started crying.

Sam and Dana walked around us and went to the cat litter box. It's a low-sided standard-size box, and there's evidence it has been disturbed; there's litter outside the box on the floor and a child's red plastic shovel in the center of the box.

"Ma'am, can you tell us how many pieces were in the box?" I asked.

With her hand nearly covering her mouth, she said, "Maybe three, four. I should have cleaned it before he got here," she admitted with guilt and sorrow.

Sam looked over at me and held up a "zero" sign with her right hand and slight grimace to go with it.

Little Skyler may have consumed three or four cat logs. This is a first for me and not sure what to even consider doing.

There isn't too much training dedicated in EMT or paramedic school that covers *litter box fudge* ingestion.

After conducting a basic exam, listening to Skyler's lungs which are clear and equal, counting a pulse on his upper arm that's at 110, he doesn't seem to be in any distress, at least at this moment.

"Ma'am, we can take him to Regional and be checked if that would make you feel better," I suggested.

"Yes, please, oh God, I'm *so* sorry, is he going to be okay?" She cried.

"Well, he looks okay. I don't see any issues right now. We'll take him to Regional and go from there," I said.

"Okay, I'll follow you in my car," she said as she handed Skyler to Rocky.

Skyler is smiling, enjoying this back-and-forth banter, and seems unfazed to it all.

We have Skyler on the gurney and headed to RGH. Dana is entertaining him with one of the many small stuffed animals we carry for just such occasions. This one an oversized kangaroo with a silly face.

Skyler is enamored with, it and we're not seeing indications he's having symptoms from the ingestion.

We don't take any transport lightly, regardless of how Skyler is acting; we're ready for any changes.

Sam placed a pediatric bag valve mask on the counter. The suction is in a ready mode. She has large towels next to the bag valve mask. We probably won't need any of this; however, if it is needed, it's usually urgently.

We're two minutes from RGH when Skyler suddenly lost his smile and had a look as if he didn't like what he was feeling.

Without warning, he vomited three times in quick successions making large piles on the gurney in front of him, each pile with chunks of the cat log pieces.

Sam immediately handed Dana one of the towels. She cleaned Skyler's mouth while rubbing his little back with empathy.

Skyler has a soured look while he's aware he tastes an unpleasant experience assaulting his palate.

After another episode and three more piles of logs, Skyler is crying. His color still looks good and breathing is okay; none the worse for the wear.

With the experience Skyler is having with this, we believe it will likely not happen again.

We arrived at RGH and his grandmother quickly showed up at the back of the ambulance as Rocky is pulling the gurney.

"Oh no, oh no," she said as she noticed the piles.

"He's doing okay, I think he got rid of all of them," I said.

We left Skyler with Sandy, a nurse, in suite 7 where he became somewhat of a celebrity after everyone hearing about his "morning breakfast of cat litter box fudge."

We headed back to the station and completed the morning vehicle and equipment checks. Strangely, we didn't seem to have an appetite until well after lunch.

Rocky was getting back into the groove after his time off. The day was kind, with Skyler being our only call well into the afternoon. It gave us time to relax and catch up on small projects around the station.

"Wow, hard to believe just two days ago Rachel and I were lying on deck enjoying the warm cloudy day, sipping margaritas," Rocky lamented.

"Well, don't forget about them EMS positions you mentioned," I suggested.

"Yeah, but my luck I'd be as busy as we are here and never get out the clinic," he conceded.

With that, the station came alive with tones resonating through the building with all of us heading to the bays.

"Rescue 41, Medic 42, respond code three for an injured male, 4400 Tamarack Street, time out 1545 hours."

Both units quickly went en route. We'd have a six-minute response. This neighborhood was very exclusive and known for its rolling hills.

"Does it feel like you just had a vacation?" I asked.

"Feels like I never left," Rocky said with a tilt of the head and re-grip of the steering wheel.

"Rescue 41, Medic 42, they are reporting the patient was run over by a lawnmower and bleeding heavily. Believed to have his arm cut off."

Steve and I both acknowledged the update.

As we turned onto Tamarack Street, a person halfway down the street is jumping up and down and waving. We're at their location within a few seconds.

The bystander ran up to my side of the ambulance and pacing nervously.

As I opened the door, he said, "Please hurry, please, he's dying."

"Okay," I said, "We'll grab our equipment and follow you."

We're led into the house and into a large kitchen area.

The patient is lying on the floor in a three-foot circle of blood at least two inches deep. He's conscious and breathing heavily. There's a female kneeling next to him who we would soon find out is his wife.

She has a large towel and working feverishly at wrapping it around his entire right arm. She has nearly as much blood on her as there is on the floor, and it's still flowing on either side of the towel.

Sam has large trauma dressings ready and knelt down next to the lady as she quickly moved to the side.

Steve carefully started removing the towel. The arm is mangled from just below the elbow to the wrist. There are shards of bone, thick layers of muscle and gaping tissue, deep purple bleeding, bright-red bleeding, and the hand is nearly severed.

It's a gruesome injury.

Steve realigned the wrist as Sam wrapped the arm with the first large trauma dressing going from the elbow to the wrist. After two additional dressings and wrapped tightly, the bleeding has stopped.

Rocky placed a cardboard splint along the lower arm with stretch gauze and lots of tape, it is secured.

Suddenly, there's a wave of calmness that has brought down the anxiety levels down, at least a few notches anyway.

The fingers of the right hand are white and waxy looking; there's obviously no blood flow beyond the injury.

The wife is intently watching and crying softly, then looking at both of her hands.

Dana has an oxygen mask over the patient's mouth and nose, and it's impossible not to notice the outright look of fear on his face.

We learned the patients name is Ted. He's thirty-seven years old. He was mowing the backyard on a riding lawnmower and tipped it over on an embankment at the end of the yard. In an instant, it was on top of him and his right arm went through the blades. He made his way to the house and collapsed on the kitchen floor, bleeding to near-death where his wife frantically grabbed the large towel trying to keep him alive until we arrived.

Kneeling next to the patient, I said, "My name is Mark, I'm a paramedic, probably a good time to head to the hospital, sound okay with you?"

Ted nodded twice and showed a hint of a smile before softly replying, "Okay, thank you."

Rocky announced, "IV is ready, I'm going to get the gurney."

"Roger that," I said.

I quickly got the rubber tourniquet over the left upper arm and miraculously found a large vein in the midarm which I put a 14 gauge into.

Considering he has no radial pulse in the left wrist, his blood pressure is dangerously low. The IV will run wide open until we get into the ambulance.

We lifted Ted and secured him on the gurney. I had a few seconds to talk to his wife as Steve and Rocky were moving Ted to the medic unit.

"Ma'am, we have things stabilized. We're taking him to RGH and we'll take care of him," I told her.

She started crying harder and she said, "Okay, okay, I'm going to get cleaned and follow you, please help him."

I put my hand on her shoulder and offered a reassuring smile and walked out to the ambulance.

We were on scene for eight minutes.

Dana has the LifePak 12 hooked up and we are seeing the first vital signs.

"Heart rate 140, blood pressure 60/34, and SpO2 won't read," Dana called out.

The first IV bag is nearly infused. Sam is switching over to the second bag.

On this one, she will place a piece of tape and write '#2' on it.

This tells the trauma folks we have infused one bag and are on the second. It's important to keep track of the amount of fluid infused during a fluid resuscitation. Too much fluid without infusing blood can be deadly.

Ted is remaining awake and still with the look of terror. Sam is up near his head and explaining everything that's going on. She's his only link to holding onto reality.

We're just about to arrive at RGH. The backdoors of the ambulance are opened as we stop and two security guards are there to help which expedited the transfer into the ED.

We're heading to suite 12. The room becomes silent while I am telling the story about the scene and care provided. Ted is headed to the OR.

For the next four hours, Ted's arm is delicately put back together. He's admitted to the trauma ICU and will have a long road to recovery. Brenda told us later they were cautiously optimistic about his prognosis.

A new day, the start of the shift and everyone is busy. From checking the ambulance cabinets, restocking, getting the medic unit washed and dried, it's a lot of work. As always, Rocky takes great pride in keeping the vehicle clean and shiny. You can have the best and most top-notched crew, but if your ambulance is dirty, that's what people see and how they judge your professionalism.

Think about it, could you imagine an ambulance showing up the way some of us keep our personal cars?

We finished and could see Brandon pulling into the station parking lot. He's been off the last two shifts and went on a mini-vacation with his new girlfriend Tara. She works in the administrative offices at the police department, and they've been dating for the last month.

They came to the station so he could give her a tour of where he works and meet the crews.

In a near-perfect chorus, we all acknowledged Brandon as he walked into the day room with Tara. This had to be a bit intimidating for her; it could get worse knowing how these things go around the station.

"Hey guys, I know everyone misses me so I thought I'd come and visit, and everyone, this is Tara," Brandon said with a large beaming grin.

This drew another collective greeting from the group which had Tara smiling and nodding to all of us.

Dana would later comment how good she felt in meeting someone shorter than she is. Tara is right at five foot, if that. Her smile makes her larger than life and she and Brandon have the look of the perfect couple.

Our social gathering took a more serious direction with Sandy's voice coming over the intercom, "Medic crew, we have a gentleman out front in a vehicle, his wife is having chest pain."

"Nice to meet you, Tara, make sure Brandon brings you here again," I said, as we all said our good-byes, Dana quickly hugging her and welcoming her to the family.

"Rocky, why don't you bring the ambulance around to the front, we'll walk out and see what we have, and put us out of service with dispatch," I said.

"Roger that," Rocky replied.

Steve, Dana, Sam, and I headed up front. Dana grabbed the LifePak 12, and Sam has the main kit. As we were going through the lobby, a middle-aged man is standing at the front door with a look of urgency.

"It's my wife, she can't breathe and the pain. We didn't know what to do. I was driving her to the hospital and she passed out, we stopped here, please, can you help her," he pleaded.

"Okay we'll go check her out, what's her name?" I asked.

"Ramona," he said. "She's sixty-two."

Rocky was pulling up as we got to the car. We couldn't see anyone in it. As we got to the passenger door, Ramona is lying across the front seat. She's blue around her lips and has an occasional loud gasp.

She's coded!

"Let's get her out of there and onto the ground," I said.

Between Steve, Dana, and Sam, we had Ramona out the car and on the ground. Dana started chest compressions, and

Sam is providing breaths with bag valve mask after Dana's thirty compressions.

Steve is cutting clothing to get the LifePak 12 hooked up. Rocky opened the kit and began setting up an IV bag and pulling medications.

"We're going to do another minute of compressions then we'll check the rhythm," I said, "When we check, Steve, you take over for Dana."

"Roger that," said Steve.

"Okay, let's check, V-fib, charge to 200," I said.

"Clear," shock delivered.

"Go for it, Steve," I said and he nodded as compressions were resumed.

"What happened here?" I wondered.

We needed history of how she got to this point. How long was she having chest pain? Did she have a history of cardiac disease?

While looking for clues, I noticed with suspicion the circumference of her left leg was considerably smaller than the right, and pale.

I found a large vein in her right midarm and put a 14 gauge into it. I handed Rocky the IV needle for a blood sugar check.

"Blood sugar is 100," Rocky announced.

"Roger that, let's check the rhythm," I said.

"Steve, stop compressions, V-fib, charge to 300 and clear," shock delivered.

Dana is resuming compressions.

"Steve, check with her husband and see what he can tell us," I said.

"Roger that," as headed into the station lobby.

I looked up as Rocky was holding a syringe of epinephrine.

"You read my mind," I said.

Rocky shrugged his shoulders as if to say, "You're welcome."

After that, it was time to intubate. Sam moved to the side and held the endotracheal tube for me.

Down the throat with the long blade and a good view of the vocal cords, "Tube please," I said.

We have a good airway, good compressions, why can't we can't get the rhythm to change?

Steve came back and explained, "Her husband says she's been bedridden over the last four weeks with a broken left leg. She got the cast off yesterday."

He then added the part I was afraid of, "She suddenly told him she couldn't breathe and started having chest pain and turned blue."

My heart sank. I think we may be looking at a pulmonary embolus. This is a clot that can develop from inactivity such as wearing a cast and being immobile for an extended period. It can travel into the pulmonary circuit (lungs) and interrupt oxygenation and cause cardiac arrest. It is very difficult to resuscitate someone who's in cardiac arrest from an embolus.

Two minutes are up and time to check the rhythm, asystole, flatline. We just went from bad to worse.

While the crew is getting Ramona loaded into the ambulance, I went into the lobby to talk to her husband.

"Hello, sir, my name is Mark, I am the paramedic in charge, we're taking Ramona to the hospital," I said.

"She's dead, isn't she?" he asked.

"Well, her heart isn't beating right now, we're giving her compressions and breathing for her," I explained.

With his head in his hands, he said, "I understand, thank you, I'll meet you guys at the hospital."

Sandy spoke up and said, "I can drive you in my car, let's go now."

I looked at Sandy, and she didn't need me to tell her this wasn't looking good.

I went to the ambulance and we're ready to go. Time for another epinephrine and we're off.

We continued the efforts to RGH where the cardiac team was standing by.

"How long have you guys been working this?" Dr. Stein asked.

"Almost thirty-five minutes," I said. And then gave the story the husband relayed to us.

"We may have a pulmonary embolus arrest here," Dr. Stein exclaimed, he then called for another rhythm check, still asystole, flatline.

After another twenty minutes of aggressive efforts, Dr. Stein looked up at the monitor and said, "Okay everyone, we're going to call it."

And that was it, Ramona was dead.

As we're leaving the room, Brenda was escorting her husband into the room. He stopped and with a vacant smile said, "Thank you for trying. She would want me to thank you for her too."

I didn't say anything. I held out my hand and during the shake I offered a hug he accepted. A couple of heartfelt pats to the shoulder and he turned to go into the room.

It never gets easier.

10

WRONG PLACE...
WRONG TIME

EVERYONE'S WALKING AROUND with a bit of soreness today. Physical fitness is an important aspect of staying healthy especially in EMS with the emotional and physical challenges. We're fortunate to have our small but adequate gym facility here in the station. We try to get some type of workout every shift.

Last shift, Sam and Dana had the bright idea of a lunges workout around the outside of the station for several laps. It got competitive and as a result we're paying for it now.

How's the saying go?

"Whatever doesn't," and that thought was stopped in midsentence by the tones.

"Rescue 41, Medic 42, respond code three for a seventy-year-old female, possible stroke, 3400 Grisham Street, time out 0831 hours."

Traffic is light and we'll have about four minutes for this response. Strokes are time sensitive for treatment and positive outcomes.

The saying in EMS for strokes is "Time is brain tissue."

This means, the quicker we get a patient into the hospital, the faster definitive treatment begins.

We're responding to an older neighborhood not without its share of problems. There are no neighborhoods completely devoid of problems; some tend to draw more attention than others.

Pulling onto Grisham Street, we see three patrol cars at the end of the street. There's a large plain-looking dark green van parked between them with the doors open and several officers standing around it. All them are holding rifles and wearing camouflage fatigues and black hoods exposing only their eyes.

As we park, I'm startled seeing Brandon walking toward the ambulance. He's wearing camouflaged pants, black T-shirt, and vest labeled with a reflective placard, "MEDIC."

"Hey guys, we had an *operation* here this morning, a bust at a nearby residence when one of the suspects bolted and ran into the patient's house. Well, the outside team followed him and about that time this little old lady came out of a bathroom, it was a dark hallway, and the guys kind of started yelling at her to get on the ground and sort of pointing rifles. Well, she collapsed and has been shaking and babbling ever since, pretty traumatic," Brandon explained.

"I tried to talk to her but she's really shook up," he added.

"Okay, thanks, Brandon, we'll check her out," I said.

How scary this must have been for her. She's having this peaceful morning and next thing she sees are these *ninjas* with big guns screaming at her.

Walking into the house, this very tiny and very anxious lady is sitting on the couch. She's rocking back and forth staring straight ahead with wide eyes and making moaning sounds in between breaths.

I slowly walk over and kneel down in front of her.

"Hi there, my name is Mark, I'm a paramedic, and can you look at me?" I asked.

No response, not even a hint of awareness. It's difficult counting a radial pulse, she's shaking so badly but its fast.

Dana made a great move by sitting next to her and putting her arm around her. The lady leaned in to her and started to cry.

I looked at Dana and gave her a suggestive look of, "Keep doing what you're doing, you're getting further than I did."

After several minutes, we're not making much progress. One of the officers handed me her ID.

Her name is Loraine. She's seventy-four years old. In the picture, she's smiling. I now know what she *should* look like.

"Loraine, can you look at me?" I asked.

With that, she looked at me, trying to speak but couldn't form the words. It was hard to watch.

With her anxiety level, I decided to give her an injection of Ativan. This is a muscle relaxer with secondary sedative effects perfect for this presentation.

Steve and Rocky brought the gurney in and we helped her onto it. Dana stayed next to her, holding her hand which Loraine was gripping very tightly by the grimace on Dana's face.

On the way to RGH, we're able to get a blood pressure.

Sam whispered to me, "170/110."

The transport continued between Loraine having episodes of crying and shaking.

Sam finally broke through with the simplest of ideas.

We carry a small collection of stuffed animals for our smaller clients. Sam selected a medium-sized gorilla with a goofy looking face, Loraine grabbed it and hugged it and started smiling. It was priceless.

We arrived at RGH. Loraine is holding her gorilla to her shoulder and petting it. Rachel escorted us to suite 4.

She looked at Loraine and softly asked, "Who's your friend there?"

Loraine looked at her and smiled, "He doesn't have a name," she said with the first hint of returning rationality.

It's difficult trying to help someone that doesn't have visible injuries. The officers on scene felt terrible about the impact this had on Loraine. Loraine will have quite the story to tell her family and friends, and how the nameless gorilla came to help her.

Back at the station, everything just stalled. There would be days like these. This is the only station in the county that has never gone an entire shift without a call.

The waiting in between calls can have added stress when you work at a busy station. You know you're going to be called; the not knowing when can take some people to the edge.

Not everyone enjoys working out of a high-call volume station. It's tough missing meals and not sleeping, every shift. All of us here enjoy the pace and couldn't imagine working at a slower station.

The afternoon began promptly after finishing lunch and kitchen cleaned with those familiar tones calling and all of us headed to the truck bays.

"Rescue 41, Medic 42 respond code three for a twenty-six–year-old male, unknown situation, the caller hung up, possibly a person not breathing, 966 Franklin Street, time out 1306 hours."

We made it out of the station quickly. We turned on 10th which would take us to Franklin and are immediately met by both lanes of traffic blocked by several people trying to push a disabled car to the side of the road.

As we pulled up, they stopped and looked back at us. One of the individuals thought we were here for them, and held his hands up yelling, "We're okay, thanks."

Rocky tweaked the siren on and off indicating we needed to get past them, and now.

Slowly they created an opening and allowed us to pass. This was a thirty-second delay we didn't need for the potential call we're headed to.

We pulled up in front of 966 Franklin and parked behind a police car.

As we walk into the house, we hear yelling from a backroom, "We're back here guys."

Down the hall and into an open room, the patient is on the floor taking slow gasps, he's purple, and the officer is giving him vigorous sternal rubs, "C'mon buddy, you need to wake up, take a breath."

"What do we got here?" I asked.

"9-1-1 advised me they got a call from an individual reporting this as a heroin OD and then disconnected the line," the officer explained.

"When I got here, the door was open and this guy's the only one in the house," he added.

"Nice to have friends, at least they called for him," I said.

"Yeah, well, he was dead purple when I first got here, after a couple of these sternal rubs, he kind of stirred and then you guys got here," the officer said.

Sam and Dana started providing breaths with the bag valve mask.

"It would be nice if we had more light in here," I said.

We had just enough to sort of see what we were doing.

Rocky handed me a rubber tourniquet, and I knelt down to look for an IV site in the left arm.

As soon as my left knee hit the carpet, I felt like I was bitten by a snake.

I knelt onto the needle and syringe the patient just used to overdose with. It not only stuck me but also it's buried to the hub sticking out of my knee.

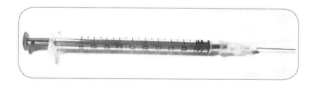

Sam tried and missed grabbing me as I rolled over onto my right side while trying to keep the needle and syringe from moving, Dana started to come to me as I raised my hand, "Keep bagging him," I said through a one-eye closed wince of shock and pain.

Rocky was at my side in an instant with his hand lightly over my chest, "Don't move," he said.

The officer looked at me and said, "Jesus, you all right, guy?"

This was bad.

Steve was bringing the gurney in when he noticed all the attention and me on my back.

"What do you need me to do?" Steve asked.

"Well, I'm going to pull this thing out, maybe you can find something to put it in, we'll bring it to the hospital with us," I said.

Steve nodded and walked out the room.

Suddenly I had a terrible thought, *Is there more?*

"Everyone, don't move, make sure there isn't any more of these around you," I announced.

Everyone looked around them and this was the only one, and I found it!

It felt like it went through the backside of my knee. In reality, it was less than an inch long, but to have a needle stab you that was just used to shoot heroin into an IV drug user was the worst thought.

AIDS, hepatitis, it all goes through your mind.

"All I could find is this plastic bowl, it has a good lid though," Steve said and handed me the container.

I pulled the syringe, placed it in the container, and ensured the lid snapped.

Back to what we came here for, I still have a patient to treat, and he isn't breathing.

I found a good vein above the left wrist. After securing the IV, we're ready for the *wake up*.

I slowly push the Narcan, and within seconds, the patient opens his eyes.

"We need you to relax, I just gave you Narcan, and you're back among the living," I said.

He looked at me, then everyone around him, then tried hard to form some response.

"What's your name?" Dana finally asked from above the patient's head.

"Ross," he said.

"Ross, do you remember what happened?" I asked.

"No, not really," he replied.

"Well, we need to take you to the hospital and make sure you're going to be okay," I said.

"I don't think I need to go, I feel okay," Ross said.

"You're going with them, partner," the officer said sternly.

"And your dirty needle just stuck him," he added while pointing at me.

Ross stared blankly with no response.

We're able to walk him into the hall and onto the gurney. During the trip to RGH we checked a blood glucose which displayed at 88.

I sat in the jump seat above the patient. I rolled my left pant leg up to check the puncture wound. There's only a trickle of blood. I wiped it with an alcohol swab, not much else to do at this point. Whatever was on the needle was already in, the instant it stuck me.

Sam watched me and offered an empathetic nod as I looked at her. It was strange, I suddenly thought, *What if it was Sam or Dana or Rocky or Steve?* I'm the one in charge on scene and would feel like I let them down.

It's a sobering moment and I'm trying to stay focused.

At RGH, Medic 42 was put out of service, I had to complete paperwork and have blood drawn. The patient refused to have his blood drawn.

My options were to have a cocktail of drugs to prevent a potential AIDS infection. Dr. Stein and I sat in his office and discussed it for a long time. He was incredibly supportive and, as busy as he was, shared his full attention ensuring I was okay mentally, I was.

He finally looked at me and said, "You were just in the wrong place, at the wrong time, my friend."

Yes I was.

EMS is an exciting world where every day is like going to a new job, but you have the advantage of already knowing how to do it. It's true. No two calls are ever exactly the same. As soon as you think you've seen it all, something comes along even more stunning and inexplicable.

This morning we came on duty and everyone's busy with vehicle and equipment checks and getting ready for whatever the day will bring.

We didn't have to wait long, it started early with the tones and spectacular-sounding dispatch.

"Rescue 41, Medic 42, respond code three for a vehicle into a house, believed to be injuries, we are getting multiple calls on this, 1224 Sycamore Street, time out 0822 hours."

We went en route and would have a four-minute response. Sycamore Street is a residential area and speed limits are very low; this wouldn't be the neighborhood we'd suspect this scenario to occur.

We're arriving in front of the address and a very chaotic scene has developed.

There are several police cars parked in front of the home. This is exactly as it sounded from the dispatch with the car completely into the front of the house. It created a large opening next to the front door, and we see the back end of the car several feet inside.

A large crowd of neighbors has assembled and watching with astonished looks. It's probably a safe guess this is the most excitement this neighborhood has had in its existence.

One of the officers would explain the intoxicated driver had been driving at a high speed when he left the road and crashed into the home. The elderly male homeowner was sitting at the breakfast table having coffee and reading the paper when the car came smashing through, hitting him, and sending him flying through a sliding glass door onto his deck.

We find an officer kneeling next to the patient who's on his right side, lying in the middle of the porch deck.

There are large menacing shards of glass on the deck along with pools of thick coagulated blood reflecting the merciless aftermath of being hurtled several feet and through the glass door.

The sliding door has small pieces of glass remaining around the edges, the dining table is overturned and the front of the car is where the table used to sit.

The patient is moaning in pain and reeling with disbelief.

"Hello, my name is Mark, I'm a paramedic, and can you tell me your name, sir?" I asked

"Buxton," he said.

"What in the Sam Hell happened?" he asked with appropriate anger.

"Well, a car came into your house and hit you," I said, and then thought about how odd that sounded.

Buxton has gaping lacerations to both arms and bleeding heavily. There's a full-thickness laceration across the forehead above both eyes with blood streaming from his face. His right leg is laterally rotated which is a classic presentation for a hip fracture. This position has his right foot turned outward and the leg is about two inches shorter than the left.

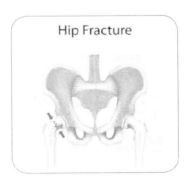

Hip Fracture

His radial pulse is 120 and he denies losing consciousness.

Sam and Dana have large trauma dressings and stopped the bleeding from the arms. Steve applied a dressing to the forehead and a stretch bandage controlling this bleeding.

He then began cutting Buxton's sweatpants and T-shirt off when he looked up at me and pointed to the right hip.

There's an outline of a hood ornament pressed clearly into the leg.

When I first looked at this, I envisioned a large blown-up photo of it being presented as "people's exhibit A" during the court proceedings and collective gasps from the jury.

Rocky has the gurney, and we're ready to secure Buxton while stabilizing his right hip. Using several pillows to support the hip, we have him on the long spine board and headed to the ambulance and transporting to RGH.

Dana is calling out the first numbers, "Heart rate at 126, blood pressure 154/94, and SpO2 at 96%," she said.

Those are good numbers considering the blood loss at the scene.

I found a good vein in the left lower arm and put a 16 gauge into it. We're two minutes from RGH and requested a full trauma team based on the (mechanism of injury) MOI and Buxton's age, eighty-four.

"I don't understand…how could a car get into my house? I'm relaxing reading the paper, and next thing I'm on the porch, how could this happen?" Buxton asked.

Sam is at Buxton's head. She opened her mouth as if she was about to answer, then realized she doesn't really have one.

We arrived at RGH and the trauma team took over. Buxton became a celebrity as the news reporters and TV stations wanted to interview him.

He was taken to the OR for his hip and admitted to the trauma ICU and expected to make a full recovery.

The driver of the car is a forty-five-year-old male. His blood alcohol level was .26, over three times the legal limit and charged with DUI and vehicular assault.

When the story went out over the news, employees from a local lumber company donated their time and boarded the front of Buxton's home. His neighbors cleaned the back porch and we're anxious to have things return to normal.

Now, we've seen it all!

11

THE SMALLER SIDE OF EMS

DANA HAS THE next couple shifts off. She's working coverage in the pediatric ICU at RGH. Nick Caffrey has the third position on Rescue 41.

"Welcome back, Nick," I said.

"Thanks, Mark, glad to be back and get the shifts," he said.

"I've been studying up on equipment if we're going to do any more 'labeling' drills," he added.

"I heard that, not funny," Sam yelled from inside the rescue.

I shrugged my shoulders and walked away.

Today was variety day, chest pain, a diabetic, a seizure, a car crash, and a child with a laceration to the head after falling out of a shopping cart. Fortunately everyone will survive and only the chest pain patient will spend the night in the hospital.

Toward the late afternoon, we're caught up on paperwork, and Nick said the dreaded magic word.

"Maybe things will 'quiet' down around here for a while," he said as everyone looked at him with shock as he dared speak the "Q word".

Not five seconds later the tones went off.

We'll need to sit down with Nick and have a serious discussion about the "do's and don'ts" around the station.

"Rescue 41, Medic 42, respond code three for a child that has fallen from a tree, 1018 Helen Place, time out 1650 hours."

The rush-hour traffic will challenge Rocky's code three driving skills getting us there quickly, and safely. Having the lights and siren can't make the traffic magically disperse; we'll be delayed by at least a minute.

Pulling up to the residence, we're met by a female, the boy's mother. She's nearly frantic and has been crying as evidenced by the smeared makeup.

"Please hurry, my son is hurt very bad, he's in the backyard, and my husband is with him," she said.

"He wanted to put him in the car, and I told him to wait for you," she added.

"Okay, show us the way," I said as we followed her around the side of the house to the backyard.

There's a massive tree at the property line. It has wood planks pounded into it for rungs that go up about fifteen feet. From there, it has a small platform that looks to be the beginning of a tree house.

At the base of it we find the patient with his father kneeling next to him and pleading for him to wake up.

"Collin, wake up, son, Collin, open your eyes, honey," he's repeating over and over.

Collin is unconscious and bleeding out of both ears. He has an obvious right femur fracture with the leg bent awkwardly and several inches in bone protruding from the midthigh.

Steve headed back to the rig for the small traction splint. This would be used to secure the right leg.

Sam went to the top of Collin's head and placed her hands over his ears providing cervical stabilization. With a fall from this height, the chances of a spinal injury could be very high.

Nick placed an oxygen mask over Collin's mouth and nose.

As I knelt down to get the initial assessment, I introduced myself and asked the father, "Can you tell me what happened?"

"I looked out the backdoor, and he was climbing the rungs. I saw him get on the platform and in the next second he was on the ground," he explained.

"All right, we're going to take care of him. If I can get you to stand back just a bit so we can help him," I said.

"Oh my God, this can't be happening," he grieved aloud as he got up.

His wife came over, and they stood near us, embracing each other as we worked on Collin.

Collin's pupils are equal and reactive. That's positive. I feel a soft spot over the back of the skull on the lower right side. He has clear and equal breath sounds over the chest. His pelvis is stable. The abdomen and upper extremities are unremarkable. His right femur is a devastating injury. He has a strong radial pulse at 110.

If Collin doesn't wake up before we make it to the ambulance, I'm going to RSI him.

Nick cut all of Collin's clothing off except the underwear.

Steve's getting the traction splint ready, and I'm going to take control of the right leg.

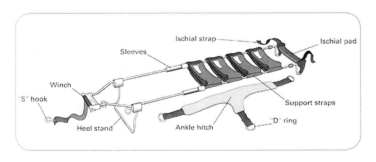

With my left hand under Collin's right ankle and my right hand behind the back of his knee, I'm ready to straighten the leg, and Steve is ready to place the splint.

Slowly, the leg is coming back in place. As I get it to proper alignment, the protruding bone has receded back under the skin.

SIGNS OF LIFE II

This isn't without inherent risk. If there's dirt or other foreign material on the bone, it can create serious complications with infection. On this injury, the bone was clean and wound is clean. It would still require careful evaluation in the ED.

Steve has the traction splint placed under his leg. Nick has the ischial or upper leg strap fastened and we're applying traction to the leg. With each click of the tensioner (winch), the leg is pulled hence the traction. When it's approximately the same length as the left leg, we'll stop. The foot has good color along with a strong pulse on the top of the foot.

Rocky has the gurney and long spine board ready and cervical collar applied.

Sam will make the call when we're ready to roll him onto the board. Nick will control the right leg during the move. Steve and Rocky will roll him toward them.

"One-two-three and roll," Sam called out from the top of Collin's head.

While he's on his left side, I check the back which doesn't reveal visible injuries or bleeding. We have him secured and ready to go.

We're on scene for nine minutes. I had Steve call RGH while we're loading Collin into the ambulance and alert them we'd need the pediatric trauma team, ETA eleven minutes.

In the ambulance, I started an IV in Collin's left midarm with a 16 gauge. We're now setting up for the RSI procedure. While I am drawing up the drugs, Nick has the LifePak 12 hooked up and calling numbers.

"Heart rate 124, blood pressure 118/64, and SpO2 at 98%," he called out.

"Roger that," I said.

"Okay everyone, stay sharp, here we go," I said.

With the drugs pushed, Collin quickly stops breathing and after sixty seconds, he's ready to be intubated.

With the laryngoscope in the left hand, I have the blade into the back of his throat and quickly find the epiglottis. A good view of the cords and after watching the tube pass into the trachea, we have Collin's airway secured.

I need to reassess. His pupils are still equal and reactive. The bleeding from the right ear has stopped. Chest sounds clear and equal. I take two more clicks on the traction splint; the legs are close to the same length now.

A femur fracture is a significant injury. There are risks to the major artery that runs along the bone; there are large muscle groups that can spasm and cause the leg to shorten. The traction splint stabilizes the bone and can prevent injury to the artery. It pulls the muscles in spasm and helps return the leg to the original length.

The spasm is a large part of the pain associated with this injury. It's one of the most painful injuries a person can endure. For new EMTs, it's a dramatic experience to see how the splint can make a huge difference in the pain. As the traction is started, the muscles are stretched and the pain suddenly goes from excruciating to manageable.

I was about to ask Nick to check the Collin's sugar when he announced, "Blood sugar is 97."

I looked at him and then at Sam displaying her innocent sly grin staring at *nothing on the ceiling*, oh well, he'll learn.

We have the usual help on the ramp of the ED and make our way to suite 12.

Collin is taken care of by the best of the best. His CT scan results show no brain injury. He has a skull fracture which will heal without invasive intervention. He's going to the OR for the femur fracture. He'll have it pinned and then to the pediatric ICU where Dana will continue his care.

Collin will make a full recovery.

Back at the station, we're all giving Nick a hard time about the infamous "Q" word. Everyone in EMS has one superstition or another, the "Q" word is unquestionably universal.

Rocky has the ambulance restocked and we're back to mission ready. We had to leave our small traction splint at the hospital and will get it tomorrow. We carry a spare just for that reason.

For the next several hours, I thought our station tones had been disconnected. We could hear the rest of the county was busy and calls were happening all around us. We weren't complaining and took the break in the action to get a nap. You couldn't depend on sleeping through the entire night. It was considered more like getting a few winks at best.

As usual, the night couldn't go without interruption; the tones had everyone heading to the bays.

"Rescue 41, Medic 42, respond code three for a four-year-old child, unknown problem, 8820 County Line Road, time out 0220 hours."

This would be the furthest response we could have within our district. It would take ten minutes.

Thoughts of what could be prompting a call for a child at this hour were swirling through my head when they were interrupted by dispatch.

"Rescue 41, Medic 42, the caller has disconnected and there's no answer on the call back, we will be advising law enforcement, 0224 hours."

Steve and I both acknowledged the update.

This was sounding suspicious and when you get those bad feelings about a call, it's not wise to ignore them.

We talk about instincts and how you develop them in EMS; they come with experience and keeping your eyes and ears open.

I tell new EMTs, "When that little voice in the back of your head is telling you something, listen to it. It knows what it's talking about and can save you and your patient. Just don't answer it aloud."

We arrived at 0229 hours. There are lights on in the house; however, no one is watching for our arrival.

Steve knocked on the front door, and after nearly thirty seconds, we're met by a male with a cigarette hanging off the right side of his mouth and holding a beer. He's wearing shorts and no shirt.

"Took you long enough," he said with the cigarette bouncing as he talked and hint of slurred speech.

"You guys live a long way out, we got here as fast as we could, what's going on tonight?" I asked.

"It's the kid, he ain't breathing right," he said.

"Okay, where is he, we'll take a look at him," I offered.

"He's in bed, sleeping," he said and turned presuming we'd follow him.

Walking through the living room, we noticed an open sliding door that led to a deck which is well lit and a large hot tub with steam rolling off it. There are several empty beer cans littered alongside it.

We continued to follow the man down a short hallway where he stopped and pointed inside a room on the left.

Walking into the child's bedroom, we find him lying on his right side atop the covers. He's wearing only underwear and they're wet, as if he'd been swimming versus incontinent (loss of bladder control).

He has a small amount of vomit next to his mouth; his breathing is irregular with occasional gurgling and gasping. His color is ashen and blue around the lips.

We're quick with the initial assessment as he has our attention with this ominous presentation.

He doesn't respond to gentle shakes to the shoulder. Sam is placing an oxygen mask over his little mouth and nose.

"How long has he been like this?" I asked.

"What do you think I am, a d——n mind reader, and what the hell's that supposed to mean?" he replied with noted annoyance.

"Hey we're here to help him, we just need to know what's going on," I explained.

"He was in the hot tub and then went to bed, that's it, *Jesus*, idiots," he exclaimed with condescension.

Nick got him on the LifePak 12 and it's showing a heart rate of 154. His SpO2 is at 82%, dangerously low. Blood pressure is 74/44. His breathing is labored at over 40 per minute. His pupils are fixed and nonreactive.

Listening to his chest with my stethoscope, I can hear fluid throughout his little lungs and suspect he may be a near-drowning patient and is in critical condition.

I need to intubate this child and take control of his airway and get him to RGH.

The father has left the room. We can hear him in the kitchen shouting incoherently while loudly opening and closing drawers. This scene is going from bad to worse to out of control, fast.

Steve got on the portable radio and requests an ETA for law enforcement.

"Be advised they're eight minutes out," was the dispatch response.

Not what we hoped to hear.

Nick then came up with a brilliant plan.

"Mark, what do think about just grabbing the child and head to the rig? We can do more there, and we'll be away from whatever this guy's issue is," he suggested.

The crew looked at me with a general consensus of accepting this plan, I nodded approval as well.

That plan was unexpectedly altered as the father came back to the room holding a steak knife and started screaming, "Get the hell out of here, now! There ain't nothing wrong with the kid," he bellowed with an enraged look about him.

He's waving the knife recklessly but not targeting any of us specifically. It's a helpless moment with consideration for crew safety and the critical condition of the little boy.

It's about to come to a climatic end, not in his favor.

Steve stood up and placed himself between the father and us, and in a calm voice said, "Sir, please, we're only trying to help your son, let us do that."

Before Steve could get another word out, the man lunged forward at him, knife first.

This was a mistake on his part as Steve was a former military police officer and hand-to-hand combat instructor.

Steve sidestepped as the man came forward. He grabbed the wrist holding the knife, and with a near-blinding move, had the man face down on the floor, right arm twisted behind him with a wristlock in place and right knee firmly planted in the small of the man's back.

Steve calmly looked up at me with a conclusive grin and said, "I think this might be a good time for Nick's plan, what do you think?"

I nodded affirmatively as Rocky grabbed the child, and Sam and I quickly exited the room as we headed to the ambulance.

Nick stayed and assisted Steve in holding the man down as he's making futile attempts to break free of Steve's grasp and howling about his arm hurting.

Once we got the child secured on the gurney, I told Rocky to go back and help Steve and Nick. Sam and I could manage for the time being.

About that time, the county deputy arrived as Rocky quickly updated him about the scenario. A few minutes later, the father was handcuffed and being escorted to the back of the patrol car.

I was able to get an 18-gauge IV established in the child's left arm. I finished drawing up the RSI drugs when Rocky and Nick made it back to the ambulance.

"Let's go ahead and get going," I said to Rocky.

"Roger that," he said, "Steve's okay and going to follow us," he added.

And with that we're headed to RGH.

The RSI were drugs pushed the child stopped breathing as anticipated. The intubation was quick, and Sam is ventilating with the bag valve.

She has her right hand squeezing the small bag valve, and her left hand is gently stroking the child's forehead above the left brow. He cannot possibly be aware of this, but if he is, it could provide some comfort to him knowing he's being taken care of, how do you know?

We arrived at RGH and there are two plainclothes county detectives holding clipboards waiting for us.

The ongoing treatment and evaluation in suite 12 was heroic as the worst fears were slowly becoming reality, the child is brain dead. All evidence pointed to a near-drowning with subsequent brain death.

The father was detained pending the investigation.

The child's name is Brady. He just turned four years old. Brady was put on life support and sent to the pediatric ICU. After twenty-four hours he would be taken off life support without regaining consciousness.

We would learn Brady's mother had been out of town helping a sick aunt and returned immediately after she was contacted.

Brady's final act in life was the ultimate gift of compassion, a life to a child in need of a heart transplant.

Brady's mother was at his side as he took his final breath. Dana was Brady's nurse and also with him at the end.

The father was charged with neglect in the death of a child and awaiting trial.

We got back to the station, it was almost 0500. It was a sobering morning. It was hard not to think of little Brady. We sat around the dining table and didn't say much.

About then the sun was shining through the kitchen window almost as if to say, "Everything will be okay."

Today is Nick's last shift on the rescue. Dana will be finished with her part-time assignment at RGH and back next shift. Of course, it's been a very slow day and calls have been minor.

We don't mind slow days or minor calls as it's just a matter of time before someone finds a way to challenge the system. Sure enough the tones were about to confirm this.

"Rescue 41, Medic 42, respond code three for an explosion, sixteen-year-old male is unconscious, 5601 Cedar Place, time out 1612 hours."

Cedar Place is on the outskirts of our district. It will take seven minutes to arrive. We can hear police scanner traffic getting reports this was a large explosion, according to the caller. We're updated with the same information from dispatch seconds later.

As we turned onto Cedar Place, there are two patrol cars in front of the residence. Neighbors are standing on the opposite side of the street staring with curiosity and sharing thoughts among each other.

As we exit the vehicles and gathering equipment, one of the deputies is walking toward us.

"Hi guys, you got a sixteen-year-old boy who just about blew himself up with some M100s. He and a bunch of friends were lighting them off, and a couple of them blew up in his hand. He's hurt pretty bad. He's around the back of the house with my partner. I'll take you to him," he said.

M100s are illegal fireworks in most areas and incredibly powerful and dangerous.

It looks like this activity has been going on for some time. There are pieces of wood, plastic, and paper scattered throughout the yard.

There are two teenagers standing next to the house on a porch with culpable expressions.

The patient is lying on the ground with one of the deputies kneeling next to him holding a towel around his left hand and against the left side of the face. The patient is moving side to side and moaning with obvious pain.

Sam and Nick are preparing large trauma dressings.

The deputy looked at me and said, "This is Kalan," while shaking his head as he got up and stepped aside.

We learned Kalan and his friends were randomly blowing things up in the yard. When they got bored with that, one of them suggested they switch to lighting M100s seeing how long they could hold them before tossing them in the air.

Kalan held two of them in his left hand, lit them both at once when one went off early. This blew a large portion of his left hand apart.

The other M100 was hurled toward his face and exploded next to his left cheek. He was unconscious for several minutes after the blast.

I knelt down and said, "Kalan, my name is Mark, I'm a paramedic. We're going to help you, we need to move the towels, and we're going to use different bandages," I explained.

Kalan moaned something we couldn't understand and continued to move back and forth in pain. As Sam removed the towel from his face, the damage is more extensive than we imagined.

His left cheek is blown open with a large crow's foot laceration. This is a pattern that resembles a crow's foot.

The left upper and lower gumline is exposed along with bleeding and bubbles coming from this horrific injury. The left side of the upper lip is shredded and this goes through the left nare. There are small shrapnel-type wounds all along the left side of the face to the hairline. A small trickle of blood is coming from the left ear canal.

The left eye is intact and I see him blinking it, the sclera (white part) is streaked with blood.

Sam placed a trauma dressing over both eyes and across the left side of the face and poured saline solution over this to cool the burns.

This is a significant injury, not only for airway issues but also cosmetically as well.

As Nick is removing the towel from the left hand the damage is equally extensive. The left thumb and index finger are attached but only as shards of bone and tissue. The palm of the hand has a deep laceration with bone, tendons, and fatty tissue exposed.

Nick placed the mutilated left index finger and left thumb to their anatomical positions and bandaged the entire hand.

Both wounds are critical. Kalan has potentially lost part of his left hand and having significant pain associated with these injuries.

While Rocky and Steve are getting the gurney ready, I'm looking for an IV site. I put a 14 gauge into a large vein in the back of Kalan's right hand.

Sam is continuing to pour small amounts of saline on both the facial and hand dressings. We have Kalan loaded onto the gurney, and he's crying out with pain.

We're now heading to RGH. Sam has placed an oxygen mask over Kalan's mouth and nose. She's leaning down near his right ear explaining what's going on and trying to offer reassurance we're doing everything we can.

With the bleeding out of his left ear, we think he may have ruptured the eardrum.

His pain level is dominating. I've given 10 mg of morphine with almost no change from his initial presentation. I've started giving him a second syringe of morphine.

"Heart rate 124, blood pressure 118/76, and SpO2 98%," Nick called out.

As long as the vital signs hold out, I can keep giving morphine. A side effect of morphine is lowered blood pressure and sometimes nausea and vomiting. The oxygen will help with any nausea.

The morphine is finally having some effect. I've given 20 mg and he's stopped moving side to side.

"Can you hear me, Kalan?" I asked.

"Uh-huh," was the slurred response and then he tried to say something else but stopped.

"We're taking you to the hospital, Kalan, just try to relax, I know it hurts, that's Sam above you," I said.

Kalan started crying softly. There wasn't anything else to say at this point. His injuries are going to change his life forever.

We arrived at RGH and went to suite 12. The trauma team gave additional morphine and removed the dressings. The injuries are extreme and graphic. Kalan is going to the OR.

He will lose the left thumb and left index finger. The facial injuries will leave permanent scarring. These are cleaned and bandaged in the OR. He's admitted to the trauma ICU and will have a long and painful recovery and adjustment to his permanent injuries. He also has an estimated 75 percent hearing loss in the left ear.

But, he is alive.

12

OUR DARKEST DAY

DANA IS BACK on shift and we're glad to see her. She brings a unique character to our station that was missed. Nick certainly proved to be a strong part of our team filling in for Dana and we're fortunate to have the people we do at Station 4.

As part of our daily ongoing training, we chose to use the time to critique our recent calls with Brady and Collin. Dana was instrumental in caring for both of them during her time at Regional, and this perspective bridged the continuation of care for all of us.

EMS can extract heavy emotional tolls on the crew with the devastating injuries and critically ill people they deal with. You wouldn't be human if it didn't have some effect on you. Having the close support network we do is vital to working through these sobering experiences and keeping everyone mentally fit.

The time was well spent; we finished our training and then had an unexpected *surprise*.

Brandon has been off for the last couple shifts and heavily involved with the SWAT team as a tactical hazardous entry medic or as his team calls him, one of "THEM." He stopped by the station seeking advice for his latest quest.

"I'm thinking about applying for a full-time position with the police department, Tara's really excited about it too," he said.

This was a shock just hearing it.

"Why would you want to leave us? Is it Dana? Did she do something?" Sam asked with a kidding curiosity.

"*What?* How do I always end up in the middle of this stuff?" Dana charged with an innocent grin.

"Oh, yeah, make a joke out of it," Brandon quickly countered, "You guys *are* my family, I could never go too far," he added.

Sam smiled and was about to speak when she was squelched by the tones calling us to the truck bays.

"Rescue 41, Medic 42, respond code three for a possible drowning, 6250 Walker Road, time out 1155 hours."

We quickly made it to the rigs and headed that way. Traffic is moderate, but we'll have an eight-minute response due to this being out in the county.

We've responded to this location before. There's a natural lake formed in a small rock quarry and it's a popular spot for the kids. It's about fifteen feet deep, and the water is fairly cold. That doesn't stop people from looking for relief during the warmer days. Today is one of them.

We have a dive team in the county, the assembling and deployment can take up to forty-five minutes. They're an all-volunteer group and respond from various locations.

We arrived and it was obvious where we're needed, the large crowd standing at the water's edge peering out to the smooth flat surface offering a grim and terrifying reality.

A teenage male came running up to the ambulance. He has jeans on and no shirt, no shoes and is dripping as if he's been swimming.

"It's a little boy, he just went under, God please hurry, I tried and can't find him," he was pleading in between sobs with arms crossed and teeth chattering.

"Okay, we'll follow you over there," I told him.

"Steve, maybe we can try to get some of those people back so we have a better idea of what we're dealing with," I said.

Steve nodded and immediately took control of the crowd.

There's an early twenties female crying hysterically and being consoled by two other females. I would learn this is the child's mother.

A witness said the two-year-old child was sitting in very shallow water just a couple feet off the bank when suddenly, he was gone. Several people have been diving and trying to find him with no success. They have the exact area the child was last seen. The pond is calm with no natural currents.

Steve immediately contacted dispatch via portable radio inquiring about the dive team and their ETA.

"Rescue 41, be advised ETA is twenty to thirty," was the unsettling response none of us wanted to hear.

Rocky looked at me and said, "I'm going in, let's get a rope from the rescue and we can tie me off."

Sam didn't give it a second thought and bolted back to the rescue for the rope.

We had no time to debate this and no better option at this exact moment. We're estimating the child has been underwater for between ten and fifteen minutes. The water is very cool at the bottom of the pond and could potentially give us an extended window in attempting resuscitation, we have to try.

Rocky went down to his boxers and T-shirt as the crowd is watching with looks of desperation and intense hope.

Steve secured the one-inch soft white rope to Rocky's right ankle. He carefully waded out a few feet and submerged.

"Dana, keep an eye on his time," I yelled out.

Dana stared intently at her watch.

After twenty seconds, Rocky came up gasping.

"It's really cold down there," he exclaimed.

After a couple of quick cleansing breaths, he went under for the second attempt.

Steve is standing at the water's edge, holding the rope with both hands, and staring intently at the point where Rocky submerged, ready to pull him to safety at the first sign of trouble.

"Thirty-five seconds," Dana yelled out.

In the next second, Rocky appeared on the surface shaking his head, nothing found. He took two more breaths and resubmerged.

Rising anxiety levels along with agonizing terror is palpable in the crowd as the seconds tick by.

Sam has the long spine board and equipment set up. She also has two blankets for Rocky in anticipation of his exit from the pond.

Suddenly, after almost forty-five seconds, Rocky bursts from beneath the surface and yells out, "I got him, give me a hand."

Steve dropped the rope and went straight into the water up to his thighs as Rocky handed him the lifeless body of the child.

He's a terrifying blue color throughout his face, eyes half open, and not breathing.

Steve places the child on the long spine board and immediately begins compressions. Dana is at the child's head with the suction unit and bag valve mask providing breaths.

The crowd has now encircled us, people are crying and, I hear the mother above them all.

Sam went to Rocky as he's slowly coming out the water. He's having trouble walking and leaning heavily on her as she's supporting him with her right arm around his waist. They make their way to the bank where she wraps a blanket over his shoulders and closes it tightly from the front, and then starts briskly rubbing his shoulders.

"Go help them, Sam, I'm okay," Rocky said and nodded, emotionally numb.

Sam went to Dana with the airway as Steve is continuing compressions. I cut the clothing away and need to find IV access. I put two rubber tourniquets on both his little arms above each elbow.

My plan is I will get him intubated and then we'll transport, continuing the resuscitative efforts en route to RGH.

As I open his little mouth, Dana is literally cheek to cheek with me peering down this small throat opening and providing suction as needed. The airway is clean; however, there are increased secretions from the stomach, Dana has them controlled and the intubation is quick and successful.

Rocky has recovered and indicated he's good to go for the drive. The child is moved to ambulance as I have a few seconds to speak to the mother.

"My name is Mark, I'm a paramedic, and we're going to take him to the hospital, we're working very hard for him," I told her.

She stared at me hanging on every word and said, "He's my baby, please," choking with emotion and covering her eyes.

A county deputy arrived and informed me he would bring her to the hospital right behind us.

We're now headed to RGH. Sam is doing compressions; Dana's providing breaths with the bag valve attached to the tube. There's good chest rise, no injuries I can find, and his color is actually looking better.

I got the LifePak 12 patches applied to his chest, and we are seeing our first rhythm.

"V-fib," I said, "I'm going to shock at 30 joules, clear," and the energy was delivered. Sam continued with compressions.

With pediatric patients, we deliver energy based on weight, in kilograms, which is roughly half your pounds weight. The recommendation is two joules per kilogram of body weight. I estimate he weighs fifteen kilograms. Subsequent shocks are delivered at four joules per kilogram.

The tourniquet I placed on the right arm yielded a vein and I'm able to get an 18 gauge established.

Dana noticed a change on the LifePak 12 and said, "Mark, we might have him back."

"Stop compressions, Sam," I said as we all looked intently at the LifePak 12 screen.

We have a good-looking rhythm, and Dana smiled as she confirmed a pulse in the upper arm.

Now to review everything and ensure we aren't missing anything.

No injuries, color is looking good, and then I get a bad feeling when I check the pupils, they're dilated (large) and nonreactive. This could be an ominous sign.

"Heart rate at 134, blood pressure 80/40, SpO2 88%, and blood sugar is 76," Sam called out.

I updated RGH and had the arrival party we expected. Moving into suite 12 and having the team take over was a tremendous relief for all of us.

I walked out the ED doors where Rocky was wringing out his shirt. Steve pulled up in the rescue and Sam and Dana joined us. We could only hope we got him to in time and done enough. This was an intense and difficult call for all of us.

"Rocky, I don't even have words, that was an incredibly brave thing you did," I said, and shook his hand and added a quick hug. He got the same from Dana, Sam, and Steve.

"Any of us would of have done it, I just thought of it first," he said humbly.

In suite 12, Dr. Stein and Dr. Leyland, the attending emergency pediatric physician, are discussing the assessment. It was solemn and heart breaking to hear as Dr. Leyland wasn't optimistic based on neurologic findings, no pupillary responses and the cardiac response was failing. You could feel the empathy as she and Dr. Stein both stared at the small child lying on the large gurney in the center of the room.

The child succumbed to the insult two hours later without regaining consciousness.

We learned his name was Dillon. His mom called him "Silly Dilly" and the newspaper had a very moving tribute we read as if we're one of our family members or close friend.

We reflected on Joe's advice of "You can't always judge your results by your efforts."

It's Friday, the last day of the month, the start of a three-day weekend and unusually warm for this time of year. Nick Caffrey is riding as a third with Rocky and I today. Once again this is a valuable opportunity for him to not only be part of the team but also further his skills and experience.

The morning vehicle check and inspection is one of the most important times of the day. Checking all the equipment and reviewing procedures pays off when you have a critical patient and the scene is moving quickly.

"I think I would like to know everything there is to know about the LifePak 12," Nick admitted to me.

"Well, be careful what you wish for, I may just assign it to you today," I said.

"And you know about the five extreme event items, don't you?" I asked.

"Hmm, I don't think I've heard of them now that you mention it," he admitted.

Sam hopped into the back of the ambulance with us when she heard the extreme event items mentioned.

"These are five items only used during extreme event-type calls," she said and then flashed me a wink.

"One is the big needle, which we carry in the main kit and on the shelf right here. It's for a tension pneumothorax and can save a life, immediately," she said with an instructive nod.

"Then there's the OB kit. It's always an extreme event if we have to deliver a baby. We carry two of them in this shelf here," she continued.

"A really extreme event is the catastrophic burn patient. So the burn sheets are critical items, they're over here in the bottom shelf," she pointed.

"Then we have probably the rarest of the extreme event items, the cricothyrotomy kit. It's in this top shelf here. This is the kit Mark can use to create a surgical airway or opening in the throat. Of course this is after all our other methods at securing an airway failed which is very rare," she said with a serious tone.

"And just a side note, our record *is* perfect for not needing this extreme event item," she added with a hint of pride.

"And the last of the extreme event items are the 10 × 30 trauma dressings. These are the largest dressings we carry and when we open one of these bad boys up, something significant has happened. We carry ten of them in this cabinet here and four in the main kit," she said.

"Now that you know the five extreme event items, you should check them every single shift when you come on duty, make sure they're there, and if you need one of them, you don't hesitate, it's strong medicine knowing your equipment, its location, and how to use it," I added.

"Wow, I thought I was just going to check some blood pressures today, not go through paramedic school," Nick said and laughed.

Steve, Dana, and Rocky are standing at the open backdoors of the ambulance, enjoying the show.

We work very hard to keep the level of care we bring to a scene the best we can offer. When I stand back and look at our crew, I have so much pride and appreciation for their unyielding dedication.

The day had an odd vibe to it in the fact we really hadn't had our normal-type shift, only two calls and one of them was a cancel. The other was a strange set of circumstances.

A thirty-five-year old female pulled into a parking garage and, in a hurry, slammed her car door shut with the right thumb, index finger, and part of the middle finger in the door and couldn't reopen it.

She fainted from the pain and shock of the incident. A bystander who happened to be parked a couple spots over noticed her sitting outside the driver's door and hanging by her trapped hand.

We arrived just after they extricated her and in time to see her faint a second time into the bystander's arms.

As Sam and Dana were splinting the hand, she passed out a third time. It became predictable she would faint if she looked at the hand or we moved it. I counted six episodes during the time she was with us, a record I cannot recall anyone coming close to. Finally, after 10 mg of morphine she became more coherent.

She had several fractures and full-thickness lacerations which needed repaired in the OR. They expect a complete recovery.

We believe there's a lesson here, don't park in a parking garage.

We are all in the day room, relaxed. The tones seemed louder and had everyone scrambling to get to the bay.

"Rescue 41, Medic 42, respond code three for an unknown situation, possible gunshot victim, 2360 Marvin Ave., time out 2115 hours."

Both units quickly went en route. Without having additional information, we could be dealing with anything and everything.

"Rescue 41, Medic 42, police are on scene requesting immediate response for a gunshot wound, the scene is secure," was the update from dispatch.

Steve and I both acknowledged the update. I looked over my left shoulder and shouted to Nick, "Stay close to me, Nick, and keep your eyes open," I said as he nodded with wide eyes.

Pulling up to the scene was difficult to sort out. There are police cars everywhere, lights flashing, people moving about with a sense of a scene gone awry.

We notice several officers waving urgently and flashlights directing us to them. We still have no idea what we're responding to but expecting the worst.

I'm in the lead, and as I walk up the driveway, there are three officers huddled next to a patient.

The first thing I noticed was the camouflaged pants. I then see the horrific pool of blood surrounding the head and neck of the patient, and officers working feverishly to control the massive wound to right side of the neck.

It was at that very second my world seemed to stop, it's Brandon.

Sam, Steve, Rocky, Dana, and Nick are also now aware of who our patient is. It feels like we're in a dream, a nightmare, but it isn't a dream, it's real.

We learned the SWAT team was conducting a search warrant for a suspected large amount of drugs and stormed the residence after breaching the front door. Brandon was the last team member through when a suspect came out of a room, and at near point-blank range, discharged a shotgun blast that caught Brandon in the right side of the neck and shoulder.

The suspect was immediately tackled and cuffed.

Brandon was dragged to the driveway where valiant efforts began trying to save him.

"Brandon, Brandon! Can you hear me? Jesus, Brandon, look at me," I called out.

There's no response; he's lost too much blood and is in and out of consciousness.

The injury is devastating. Brandon has a large portion of the right side of the neck shredded and several smaller holes at the right clavicle. The bleeding is catastrophic. He's ghostly pale, struggling to breathe. His skin is so cold.

Sam and Dana both have large trauma dressings and have the wound packed. Rocky has the gurney behind us, and as I make eye contact with him he tosses me two rubber tourniquets. I put one on each of Brandon's arms above the elbow.

Nick has an oxygen mask and holding it over Brandon's mouth and nose. Steve finished cutting Brandon's clothing, and we're ready to lift him to the gurney.

We are on scene four minutes.

I can feel the ambulance accelerate as Rocky has us moving toward RGH. Nick has the LifePak 12 hooked up.

"Heart rate 136, blood pressure 60/32, and SpO2 doesn't read," Nick called out.

Sam is actively crying as she's setting up an IV bag.

I notice a large vein in his left midarm and put a 14 gauge into it. I'm going to RSI Brandon. With the drugs drawn up, I push them through the IV line. Within seconds, Brandon lets out an exhaustive breath and is ready for the intubation.

Despite the catastrophic wound, the intubation is without complication. Dana is now ventilating Brandon with the bag valve. She's focused on getting every breath in with a steady stream of tears coming from both her eyes.

"Mark, look at the monitor," Nick called out.

The heart rate has begun to slow down, 80-65-44-20-10, flatline. I watched Brandon's final beat of life go across the screen. Brandon just coded.

Nick began compressions as I was updating RGH. We'll be there in two minutes.

We arrived to an army of help and made it into suite 12. A trauma surgeon began aggressively exploring the neck wound looking for something to stop. There wasn't anything, Brandon had bled out.

Twenty minutes after we arrived, the efforts were halted. Brandon was pronounced dead.

We're in shock, crying and hugging, Sam collapsed against the wall with her hands over her face, Dana grabbed her, and Sam buried her face against Dana's neck.

Joe was contacted and arrived several minutes later. He informed me we'd be out of service the rest of the shift. We couldn't run another call if we wanted to anyway.

We gathered in the EMS break room. This is unprecedented territory for us, all of us. We deal with death and have never had to "deal" with it.

I went outside and walked around the ambulance several times like I was lost, then back to the EMS break room.

Everyone is reliving the scene over and over in their minds.

I finally broke the silence. I had to let everyone know.

"He knew...he knew it was us," I said and had everyone staring at me.

"When I, when I first got to him, I called his name, he didn't answer, I looked away for a second, and then felt like I needed to look back, he was looking at me, he blinked twice and that was it," I explained.

"He knew it was us taking care of him, he knew he wasn't alone," I said and put my head in my hands and just sat there.

Brandon was thirty-five years old. He submitted his application to the police department earlier that day. He was single and an uncle to his brother's ten-year-old son, and Tara's boyfriend.

The county provided us two additional shifts off. We all attended Brandon's service and it still doesn't seem real, but life will go on.

If Brandon could somehow give us some advice, we believe he would say, "Don't stop what you guys do, it's too important, and we always believed we could make a difference, keep going!"

13

ALTERNATIVE MEDICINE

IT'S TOUGH GOING through the stages of death and dying after losing a friend or coworker and in the manner which took place. We're part of it regularly within the scope of our profession, but aren't personally involved with it as we are now. We're getting better, the last couple days have been a little easier, and the path leading us to an acceptance seems clearer.

Dana has become good friends with Tara. Tara hasn't been back to work and is having a difficult time with the loss of Brandon. Dana brought her to the station, and we've gotten to know her a little better. We can see what Brandon saw in her; she's caring, funny, and knows we still consider her part of our extended family.

We've been back to work for a few shifts, and the start of the day is with a breakfast second to none, courtesy of Steve. It's the works, pancakes, waffles, eggs. Now everyone needs a nap.

The morning pretty much flew by with only two calls. The last one seemed to take forever.

We responded for an elderly lady with pneumonia who was going to be admitted to RGH. Only problem was she lived alone and wouldn't leave the house until we found a sitter for her beagle, Lulu.

The poor little dog wouldn't leave her side. All through our exam and treatment, Lulu sat there as if to approve or disapprove of the procedure. When I started the IV, Lulu gave me a subtle growl and sideways leer.

We finally got in touch with her daughter and she came to sit with Lulu. As we left, Rocky noticed Lulu standing on the back of the couch, staring out the large picture window watching the ambulance leave.

We're setting the training room up. We have several mannequins we use for various difficult airway scenarios and can be intubated or simply managed with a bag valve mask.

This is important training as it pays off when we're faced with difficult airways.

In reality, there's no such thing as an "easy airway." You have to be proficient at every aspect of creating and maintaining an open airway and it can be humbling.

One of our volunteer EMTs came to me last week and wanted a recommendation for paramedic school. I applauded him for his aspiration in this goal.

I asked him, "How many airways have you established by yourself and tell me about some tough ones you had?"

He looked at me for several seconds like I punched him in the gut.

"Those are EMT skills," I explained. "When you go to paramedic school, you better pretty much be an expert on the basic airway skills," I added.

"Always remember this, the *best* paramedics were the *best* EMTs," I told him.

He shook my hand and said, "Do you mind having a rider now and then?"

"Anytime, my friend, anytime," I said.

Our airway training class would have to be put on hold; the tones had other plans for us this afternoon.

"Rescue 41, Medic 42, respond code three for an unconscious forty-four-year-old male, possible overdose, 214 Orchard Hill Circle, time out 1323 hours."

Both crews went en route quickly and traffic was unusually heavy. We would still have a short response.

A police officer is arriving just as we pulled in front of the residence. The police presence ensured the crew's safety as things didn't always go without incident on overdose scenes.

Last month, a crew from a neighboring station responded to a heroin OD and ended up in a fight that put one of them in the hospital overnight with a concussion. No call is ever *routine.*

A female answered the door with a paranoid look about her and asking us to hurry. The officer is through the door first followed by the rest of us. There are several individuals sitting in the living room. They all have the same paranoid look the female has and none of them are making eye contact, very creepy.

"He's in the bathroom," she said.

"Okay, show us the way," I said. "What did he overdose on?"

"Like I'm going to tell you with him here," she said and glared at the officer with subtle contempt.

I looked at the officer as we shared a grin.

It really isn't critical to know what the patient took in the first few minutes of the call. We'll prioritize our treatment to ensure the ABCs (Airway, Breathing, and Circulation-pulse) are intact and then we look for specific characteristics.

Narcotic overdoses are classic with the decreased respiratory effort and pinpoint pupil presentation.

Walking into the bathroom, we find the patient fully clothed and sitting in the empty bath tub. His shirt and pants are wet and he has circumoral cyanosis (blueness around the lips and mouth) with his eyes half closed. About then he takes a large gasp and then back to nothing.

"Let's get him out the tub and start bagging him," I said.

"Roger that," Steve said, and between him and Sam the patient was quickly on the floor.

During the lift out the tub, several ice cubes fell from his pants and shirt.

This was a common practice used in the sixties and seventies by junkies trying to shock the patient into waking up. It has no real therapeutic effect other than being really cold but every now and then we still see it attempted.

Dana has the bag valve mask and began giving breaths.

"Pupils are pinpoint," she called out.

This guy has absolutely no veins I could find other than the big one on the left side of his neck. So in goes the 14 gauge.

We're now ready to wake him up.

The Narcan is pushed slowly, and within seconds his eyes open fully and the ubiquitous surprised look.

"Welcome back," I said, "can you tell us your name?"

"Kelly," he said.

"Okay, Kelly, do you know why we're all here in the bathroom with you?" I said.

"No," he said.

"What do think about us taking you to the hospital," I said.

"No thanks…I'm okay," he said.

"Well, the Narcan we gave you won't last as long as the heroin in your system," I explained.

"I didn't do any heroin," he quietly protested.

I got down close to his ear and whispered, "Look, Kelly, I know you did the heroin, you know you did the heroin, my Narcan that woke you up knows you did the heroin, so we have to take you to RGH, and you can tell them what you want or don't want."

"It's not fair, man," he said.

"Well, let's go, can you walk?" I said.

And with that he was up and walked into the living room where Rocky has the gurney waiting. The visitors sat around as if we weren't there, staring straight ahead and just nothing, still very creepy.

During the transport to RGH, Sam was asking Kelly questions for the medical report when he just stopped talking. He gave a loud gasp and that was it, out again. We lowered the head of the gurney, and Sam got ready to start bagging with the bag valve mask. I quickly opened a box of Narcan, pushed half of it slowly and Kelly sprung to life again.

We didn't tell him what just happened. I doubt he would have believed us.

At RGH we went to suite 7 where Rachel took the report.

"How did his pants and shirt get all wet?" she asked.

"That's where the ice cubes melted, of course," I said.

Rachel smiled and winked.

We made it back to the station at 1530 hours. One of the Station 4 volunteers brought a small platter of treats for the crew. We had cake, cookies, candy, and a gallon of milk. One thing we couldn't complain about was more often than not we had some type of *appreciation food* being brought to the station. We'd say we really shouldn't be indulging but somehow it all seemed to disappear before the end of the shift.

Rocky gave us an interesting update after talking to Rachel. Kelly needed a third dose of Narcan and was being admitted for observation. If we'd have left him home as he preferred, he may not have survived.

After filling up on goodies and getting the medic unit restocked *and* washed for the second time today, we're listening to the tones calling.

"Rescue 41, Medic 41, respond code three for a gunshot victim, 9346 Davidson Road, time out 1622 hours."

We'd have at least an eight-minute response time. Davidson Road was a rural address and not too many calls to this area.

"Rescue 41, Medic 42, be advised that law enforcement is responding, ETA four minutes, the patient has been shot in the abdomen with a shotgun, he is conscious at this time."

Steve and I both acknowledged the updated information. It was important to know how far out law enforcement would be. We couldn't arrive on scene before it was safe to do so. Not knowing the circumstances of the incident could potentially place the crew in the middle of a dangerous situation.

We're just a couple minutes from the scene when dispatch gave the clearance to respond directly to the scene.

The residence has a long driveway leading to the house. As we pulled up, we're met by one of the deputies. He's advising the patient is in the back of the residence on the deck.

We see a male in the back of one of the patrol cars, and he's staring blankly ahead. He doesn't look at us as we walk past.

Walking around the side of the house, we go up several steps to the deck. We find the patient lying on his right side and another deputy holding a large towel to the lower left abdominal area.

We would learn through the course of getting this scene handled, the patient is eighteen years old and his name is Scott. Him and his older brother (the one in the police car) had been drinking all day and reportedly consumed a case of beer each. At some point, they began fighting and Scott got the best of his brother.

The brother went into the house and retrieved a 12 gauge shotgun. He came outside pointing the gun where Scott looked at him and dared him to do it, in the next instant he was shot once through the lower left abdomen.

Scott is lying in a large pool of blood and tissue and crying with obvious pain. The wall behind him has the remnants of where the shot passed through his side. He didn't take the blast directly to the abdomen or he'd have certainly been killed outright.

Sam and Dana have large trauma dressings and are ready to take over from the deputy.

I knelt down next to Scott and put my hand on his left shoulder, "My name is Mark, I'm a paramedic, and we're going to take you to the hospital, do you understand me?" I asked.

I'm checking his radial pulse at the same time, and it's 120 beats a minute.

"Uh-huh, he shot me, I didn't do nothing," he said while reeling from the intensity of the assault.

As we pulled the towel away from the wound, the damage is extensive. The concentration of the blast was just above the beltline on the left lower side. Pellets have penetrated up along the left lateral chest and down to the left groin region and fortunately missing the vital area.

This wound has a tremendous potential for catastrophic internal bleeding from bowel, left kidney, spleen, lung, and other vascular-rich structures in this pathway.

Steve has the clothing cut away except for the bits of shirt imbedded within the wound, and Rocky is coming around the corner with the gurney and long spine board.

Sam and Dana do an excellent job of packing the abdominal hole left by the blast. They secured the dressings with stretch gauze encircling his lower abdomen.

A quick listen to breath sounds reveals decreased air movement on the left side. The pellets have obviously collapsed some lung fields. None of the entry wounds are bubbling, which means I may have to insert the big needle into his left chest to relieve the air pressure if it becomes a tension pneumothorax.

Dana has an oxygen mask over his mouth and nose.

We'll secure him with full spinal precautions as we don't know where all the pellets ended up. They could have traveled into the spine.

As we're moving to the ambulance, I am paying close attention to Scott's respiratory pattern. He's becoming more agitated and working harder to breathe. He's developing a tension pneumothorax. His left chest is building pressure and starting to affect the function of his good lung on the right side.

Left untreated, he will die from this.

I jump into the back of the ambulance ahead of them as they are loading the gurney. I have the big needle out and ready.

I map out the landmarks, midclavicle, between the second and third ribs, and insert the needle.

Scott screams out in pain as it penetrates the skin.

In the perfect world, it might be worth injecting a small amount of numbing agent where the needle would be inserted. If we had this kind of time, then we wouldn't need it in the first place.

Seconds later it's hissing like an open air line and becomes silent. Scott is breathing fast, but not as labored.

We're now en route to the hospital. I need to get at least two IVs started. I apply rubber tourniquets to both upper arms. The first vein I see pop up is in the right midarm. I put a 14 gauge into it and tape it securely. We cannot afford to lose this line.

Dana has the LifePak 12 hooked up and calling out numbers.

"Heart rate 126, blood pressure 76/42, and SpO2 isn't reading," she said.

With his low SpO2 readings, I'm making a decision to put Scott asleep and RSI him. This will allow us to provide a higher level of oxygenation and monitor and control his airway closer.

As I am preparing the drugs, Dana calls out, "Heart rate is now 134…blood pressure is 66/40."

Scott is bleeding out and we need him in the OR.

I push the etomidate through the IV line and Scott rapidly goes to sleep. Then the sux, and his breathing has stopped, he's ready for the intubation.

Slowly, the laryngoscope blade goes into the back of his throat. The alcohol fumes are overwhelming. I have a good view of the vocal cords and pass the endotracheal tube.

After the first couple of breaths with the bag valve, we notice sprays of blood coming up the tube from the lungs. We also have blood coming through the chest needle. Scott may be losing more blood in the chest cavity than through the abdominal blast.

I found another vein in the back of the left hand and put an 18 gauge into it and now have two bags flowing wide open.

"Give us something to work with here, Scott, hang on," I whispered aloud.

"Heart rate 128, blood pressure 72/44, and SpO2 86%," Dana called out.

"Thanks, Dana," I said noting they are *slightly* better.

We are now just minutes from RGH.

Pulling up to RGH was a relief. Knowing Scott needed to be in the OR versus the back of our ambulance is an uneasy feeling. Trying to move faster than time allows is frustrating in EMS.

Dr. Aston is the chief trauma surgeon for RGH and in charge of the resuscitation from here out. The room is listening and working at the same time as I relay the story of what unfolded here this afternoon.

As I finish my story, Dr. Aston secured a chest tube to the left chest with blood immediately filling the drainage tube.

I'm leaning against the counter watching everything unfold.

It's a choreograph of activity nothing short of perfection, each member of the team skillfully moving about and preparing Scott to move to the OR.

I left the room and walked through the automatic doors to the ED entrance. Rocky, Sam, and Dana are cleaning the back of the ambulance.

There's blood on the floor, torn packages, equipment everywhere, and the oxygen port on the wall is still hissing.

This is our office, a mobile intensive care unit, one of the most intense-working offices on the planet. Very few people would be comfortable here, or understand why we are; we wouldn't be content anywhere else.

Scott made it into the OR, and after several hours of surgery, he's admitted to the trauma ICU in critical but stable condition.

He's lying in the ICU fighting for his life while his brother is sitting in a jail cell, both of their lives changed forever in an instant.

This morning, coming on shift is the start of major projects we need to complete around the station. The inventory for the ambulance needs updated and drug expiration dates checked. We're also cleaning the compartments which we try to do monthly. They get dusty and it's easier to accomplish this during the inventory.

After a planning meeting in the kitchen over coffee and donuts courtesy of Sandy, we're ready to get started.

As most days go, projects would take a second seat to the tones coming across the ceiling speakers loud and clear ensuring we don't miss them.

"Rescue 41, Medic 42, respond for a male in seizure, 180 Douglas Street, in the backyard, time out 0943 hours.

This will be a quick response, no more than two minutes with rush-hour traffic pretty much over.

We pulled up in front of the residence, and a male is walking from around the back of the house toward us. He's waving a couple times and I acknowledged him.

"Hi, guys, thanks for coming, I think I got him doing okay now," he said.

"Okay, well my name is Mark, I'm a paramedic, what do you have going on?" I asked.

Sam, Dana, and Steve have collected our kits, and we're following the male around the back of the house as he's explaining the story.

"Well, it's my friend, I'll be honest, we been drinking a little this morning, he just fell over and started having another seizure," he explained.

"All right, has he ever done this before?" I asked.

"Oh hell, he drinks every morning," he said and chuckled.

"Well, I meant the seizure, has he ever had those before?" I asked.

"I told you, man, he has them seizures all the time, this one seemed worse though," he said.

"What do you mean by *worse*?" I asked.

"Well, he was gagging so I had to fix him, like an emergency-type deal and keep him from swallowing his tongue," he explained.

We make it around the back of the house and the patient is lying under a tree.

"Is that a stick, sticking out his mouth?" I turned and asked Rocky.

"No, it looks more like the whole branch," he replied.

The male would go on to describe how this two-inch round tree branch was all he could find to shove in the friends mouth in order for the tongue to be saved from being swallowed.

He's very proud of this deed and repeats it several times.

Sam and Dana immediately go to the patient's head, Sam gently pulls on the branch, and it freely comes out the mouth.

The patient is blue, eyes are half closed, and he has tree shavings and dirt throughout the inside his mouth. His tongue is lacerated creating a small pool of blood to collect which causes him to start gagging and coughing violently. This causes Dana and Sam to raise the *instinctive* arm as to protect them from the bloody spray.

Then he begins seizing, grand mal in nature, which lasts for sixty seconds. During this activity, Sam is protecting his head from slamming on the ground, and Dana is suctioning as needed.

Rocky has the kit open and set up for an IV. Steve is supporting the patient, who has been placed on his left side, as the seizure starts to wane.

Dana secures an oxygen mask to his mouth and nose. Sam is providing a jaw thrust maneuver, and we're seeing good breaths being taken.

After applying the rubber tourniquet to the right arm above the elbow, I place a 14 gauge in the midarm.

Steve has the LifePak 12 hooked up and calling numbers, "Heart rate at 114, blood pressure 108/66, and SpO2 at 84%," he said.

"Sugar at 92," Rocky called out.

"Roger that," I said, let's get ready to load and go, we can finish this in the ambulance.

With the patient on his left side and secured on the gurney, we're heading to RGH.

"How's the secretions and bleeding?" I asked Dana.

"They've slowed, and he's actually breathing okay now, I can see him opening his eyes occasionally," she said.

"Okay, sounds good," I said.

I got down to the patient's face and said, "Hey there, can you open your eyes for me?"

He slowly opened them and looked around.

"Where am I?" he asked.

"You're in the ambulance, you had a seizure," I explained.

"Again, damn it," he said.

"Do you hurt anywhere?" I asked.

"My mouth feels dry and my tongue hurts," he said and sticks it out trying to look at it.

I'm sure it does, I thought.

We arrived at RGH and were directed to suite 4. Rachel is working, and I gave her the report as she stood with mouth agape wondering how much of this really happened.

The patients name is Charley, he's forty-four years old. His blood alcohol is .33, over four times the legal limit. He was admitted for twenty-four hours and discharged the next day.

Despite his friend's attempt to knock him off, he would survive to drink another day.

14

ONLY IN OUR WORLD

Our involvement with the community goes beyond responding to 9-1-1 calls. We're occasionally invited to schools around graduation to discuss the dangers associated with drinking and driving or equally dangerous cell phone use and texting while driving. This is presented as coming from an impact perspective in the prehospital view.

We've also participated with the health classes as they complete their first aid or CPR training.

Today, Rocky and I will be evaluators for CPR practical testing in Mrs. Craven's class of juniors and seniors.

We split up to evaluate two different practical stations, and if this is an example of the future for EMS, we're in very good hands. The students excelled with competence and enthusiasm.

With time at the end of the class, as always, they want to hear the stories, the tragedies, and the gore. Everything is exciting at this age with no perceived vulnerabilities. What they cannot appreciate is the *naiveties* they have, sometimes with dramatic life-changing consequences.

We see examples day in and day out of risky activity and terrible choices we'd enjoy sharing with teens that are vulnerable and still at malleable ages.

We were discussing this back at the station when the tones fit right into the conversation.

"Rescue 41, Medic 42, respond code three for an unknown medical problem, unconscious person at the Shoppers Outlet, 2300 Powell Street, time out 1042 hours."

We followed the rescue as they made it out the bay first. We should be there in less than four minutes even with the midmorning traffic congestion.

Most drivers are courteous and try to give us the right of way during code three driving, lights, and siren. There's a small group with no regard for yielding any part of the road they evidently "own."

We've actually had people cut us off from making a turn or driving in a manner not allowing us to go around them. Of course, there's never a police officer around when this happens.

The Shoppers Outlet is a massive grocery warehouse and several small food courts located throughout the store. It's always busy.

We parked directly in front of the store, people everywhere as usual. A young courtesy clerk met us at the door with an anxious and worried look.

"She's in one of the bathrooms. I think she might be dead," the clerk said.

"Okay, lead the way, and we'll follow you," I said.

We walked into the store and drew hard stares and concerned looks from the shoppers. This reaction was always the same. Even if we're in the store picking up an item for the station we'd get the once-over.

"Anything else you can tell me about what's going on?" I asked the clerk.

"Well, one of the customers came to the office and told us a lady was snoring in the bathroom. When the manager went to check, her face was blue, and she looked *dead*," she said with a grimace.

I looked at Rocky with raised eyebrows and mouthed the word, "WOW."

We made it to the bathroom, the door is propped open, and several bystanders have gathered watching the incident play out.

The patient is a small-framed, late twenties female, crumpled awkwardly in a stall. She's cyanotic (blue); not breathing and then I notice a syringe lying on the floor beside the toilet.

"Let's get her out of here kind of fast guys, Sam, you and Dana get ready with the BVM," I said.

Just as Steve and Rocky started to lift her, she began convulsing quite violently. This went on for several seconds before they could reestablish their grips and lift her to the open floor.

One of the main causes for convulsing, or seizure, is hypoxia or lack of oxygen. As the brain becomes more and more oxygen deprived, it responds with irritation and firing signals wildly which causes the seizure. Treatment is aimed at correcting the underlying problem, in this case, the hypoxia.

She's wearing high-thigh jean shorts, a long sleeve black thin sweater, and flip-flops. The left one has fallen off. Her left sleeve is rolled up above the elbow, and there are several bruised areas along the vein tracks on the left lower arm.

Her face is now nearly a blackish purple. She has vomit down the front of her sweater, blood and secretions coming from her mouth and pupils are pinpoint.

After clearing her mouth with the towel from the gurney, Sam has the mask positioned over her mouth and nose, and Dana is squeezing the bag. We can see good chest rise and fall.

Rocky has the kit open and setting up an IV bag and has the glucometer ready.

Steve is cutting the black sweater off and preparing to hook up the LifePak 12. He suddenly pauses with a puzzled expression that isn't characteristic of him.

She isn't wearing a bra, and each nipple is pierced with a thick gold post and then a gold chain attached from post to post. Steve managed to work around the chain, place the electrodes and cover her with the cut-up sweater.

"Heart rate 136, blood pressure 96/54, and SpO2 at 84%," Steve called out without looking up as he usually does.

"Roger that," I said.

After applying the rubber tourniquet to the right arm above the elbow, I'm surprised to see the vein pop up on her hand. An 18 gauge went right with no problem.

"Glucose is 166," Rocky announced.

"Roger that, 166," I repeated.

We're ready for the Narcan. Steve will control the lower extremities in case of aggression, and Rocky, Sam, and Dana are ready to roll her if she starts vomiting again.

Within seconds of the Narcan going through the IV line and into her vein, she opens her eyes. It takes several more seconds and some heavy blinks before she responds.

"Where am I?" she asked in a bewildered fog of confusion.

"You're in the Shoppers Outlet bathroom," I informed her.

"Can you tell us what happened today?" I asked.

"I don't know, I don't feel good," she said.

"Well, my name is Mark, I'm a paramedic, I think you might have OD'd," I told her.

"Ahh man, no way, please, please just let me go, man, I'm okay," she said.

"Can you tell me your name?" I asked her.

"Serena," she said.

"Okay, Serena, here's what we have to do, you need to be evaluated at Regional. If they don't have any problems with you going home, then you can leave," I said.

"Do you hurt anywhere?" I added.

"No, man, I just feel really sick," she said.

"Dana and Sam will help you on the gurney, and we'll see if we can get you feeling better in the ambulance," I told her.

With Serena covered in a secured and reclined sitting position, we started to wheel her out the bathroom. By now the curiosity crowd has grown. Many of them would regret that urge to watch after what followed next.

Serena suddenly leaned over to her left, toward the crowd, and began violently projectile vomiting. It was coming out in torrential streams splattering loudly on the shiny linoleum floor, and then the warm offensive aromatic wave crept out to the crowd.

I was surprised we didn't end with a patient from the observation galley, especially the ones with the best seats in the front row.

We're parked in front of the store in the fire lane. It's marked with obvious red paint along the curb and large sign. There's a minivan parked directly in front of the ambulance and no driver in it.

After getting the gurney secured into the ambulance, Steve had to stop people from exiting the store as Rocky backed up in order to get around the minivan.

The transport is uneventful; we arrived at RGH and delivered Serena to Rachel with a full report.

Serena was discharged four hours later and we haven't seen her again.

Finally back to the station and time for a late lunch. Steve came into the kitchen with the rest of the parked minivan story.

"The driver came out after you guys left pushing a small cart of groceries. I informed her she was blocking the ambulance, and she argued it was a fire lane, not an ambulance lane, thus she wasn't breaking any laws blocking it," he explained.

"Did you ask her where she kept the hoses on her minipumper?" Rocky asked.

"No, I just looked at her for several seconds with a dumb look on my face," and then said, "Oh, well that makes perfect sense, and have a nice day."

In EMS, every call has the potential to go completely sideways at any given time. Welcome to our world.

Nick Caffrey had been filling in as Joe's partner on Medic 41 since Brandon's murder. Joe was deeply affected by Brandon's death as we all have. Joe and Brandon were partners for almost ten years. That's a long time and you get to know your partner very well in EMS.

Nick was hired on full time in the EMT driver position on Medic 41 today. There was no fanfare other than us welcoming him to the station and ensuring he understood we're all here together, one team.

Nick is married to Veronica "Ronnie" who's a bank manager, and they have two small daughters.

The slow pace of the day is interrupted with a chilling dispatch coming after the tones.

"Rescue 41, Medic 42, respond code three for a twenty-eight-year-old male patient trapped underneath a vehicle, 1630 Utah Street, time out 1440 hours."

Both crews were moving quickly at the sound of this incident. Every second he's trapped could lower the odds of a successful outcome, if he was even still alive.

We've responded to devastating outcomes during "backyard mechanics gone wrong."

Several months ago, we were dispatched as we came on shift for a possible DOA in the back of a residence. The call was generated by a paper delivery boy who happened to notice the patient lying under a flattened vehicle and not moving.

We arrived and used air bags to raise the vehicle. The patient had been working under it when it slipped off the jack killing him instantly with a massive crushing head injury. He was seen by neighbors the previous afternoon working on the car and had gone unnoticed.

This response would take three minutes. Rescue 41 has air bags that can lift a car with ease. Steve would be responsible for this once we arrived if the patient was still trapped. They carry several of these specialized air bags, and each one is capable of quickly lifting thousands of pounds.

"Rescue 41, Medic 42, be advised the patient has been extricated by bystanders, he is unconscious at this time with difficulty breathing."

Steve and I both acknowledged the update.

As we pulled onto Utah Street, we immediately see two females frantically waving in front of a residence. Before Rocky could bring the ambulance to a stop, they're running to us with off the charts anxiety levels.

I open my door and they start talking trying to explain what happened and none of it's making sense in their panicked state. We grab the gear and follow them toward an open garage.

There's a car backed into the garage undergoing obvious restoration of some type and jacked up on the driver side. Both front tires are removed and wood blocks are scattered over the concrete beneath the car.

Two guys are kneeling next to the patient a few feet away from the car.

One of them is shouting, "Breathe, Jeff, c'mon, man, breathe, take some breaths."

We would learn Jeff was under the middle of the car when it shifted and fell off the blocks, the weight of car pinned him from the midchest and head for several agonizing minutes.

The friends quickly got the jack under the driver's side and were able to drag him free after raising the car. He was described as initially being a black purple from the neck up and not breathing. Since then, he's been unresponsive and having gasping attempts to get a breath.

Jeff has massive injuries. His color alone is frightening with a deep purple through his neck, lips, and most of his face.

This is traumatic asphyxia. It occurs when the chest is compressed and blood flow back to the heart is compromised. The patient gets profoundly hypoxic and it can carry a high mortality rate.

The right side of his face is deeply lacerated with a gaping wound going from the chin to the cheek. The right eye is tightly closed with deformity noted to the lower socket. He's also bleeding from the right ear canal. The left eye is bloodshot but the pupil is reactive.

Dana is cutting clothing and exposing the chest with major findings.

The right side is sunken in above the nipple line, and air is felt under the skin, the rice krispies.

He does have a carotid pulse which I placed an "X" over with my pen.

Steve and Sam have the bag valve mask out. When Sam squeezes the bag we cannot see chest rise. Jeff will need to have his airway secured by RSI procedure.

Dana is applying a dressing over the gaping right face laceration and eye. A stretch bandage will hold it secure.

Rocky has the long spine board in place. I'm placing a rubber tourniquet on each upper arm in hopes of having a vein to select in the ambulance.

We roll Jeff onto his left side as we slide the spine board in behind him. We always roll the patient onto their *good* side as to not aggravate the injury. The procedure goes quickly and we're headed to the ambulance.

I have a few seconds to talk to the group in the garage. One of the females is Jeff's wife. The two men and other female are friends.

"Is he going to be okay?" his wife asked pleadingly.

"Well, he has some very serious injuries. We're doing everything we can and we're taking him to Regional," I said.

With that, she started crying and had to be assisted into a chair.

"We'll bring her to the hospital," one of the friends said.

I put my hand on her left shoulder and said, "We'll take care of him," and turned toward the ambulance.

As I jumped into the back of the ambulance, I could see Sam using the suction to clear the airway of foamy blood filling the back of Jeff's throat.

I needed an IV in quickly to get his airway secured. There's a large vein in the left midarm and I put a 14 gauge into it. Now the LifePak 12 so we can see what's going on inside the chest.

The heart rate is 124, the blood pressure 70/40, and the SpO2 sensor is reading 78%. These are poor first numbers.

Dana called out, "Mark, this bagging is getting tougher. I think we may need to needle the chest."

After a quick reassessment of the chest, Dana is correct, there's no air movement on the right side, a classic tension pneumothorax accompanied with his degree of distress and failing vital signs.

The landmarks are difficult to map out with the injuries. Doing the best I could, the big needle is inserted with an immediate hiss for several seconds followed by oozing and bubbling blood.

This is all part of the pathophysiology of traumatic asphyxia. The lung tissue itself is bruised and bleeding; thus, producing the foam as the big needle is inserted. It's also the reason the SpO2 is so low; the tissues where oxygen exchange takes place is injured. It is a vicious cycle.

The RSI drugs are drawn up and everyone's in place. Dana pushed the etomidate with immediate effect noted followed by the sux. Jeff is now paralyzed and not breathing for at least the next four to eight minutes.

With the laryngoscope in my left hand, I make my way to the back of the throat. Sam is suctioning as I call for it. It's unsettling seeing bloody foam coming up through the trachea.

Then the clear view of the vocal cords and watching the tube go into the trachea.

Dana has the bag valve attached to the tube. With the first squeeze of the bag, we can see good chest rise. We're still seeing the blood-tinged foam coming up through the tube.

"Hear rate 128, blood pressure 74/34, and SpO2 at 86%," Sam called out.

This is still bad but better than they were initially.

I found another good vein in the lower part of the left arm and put a 14 gauge into it. We now have two good IV lines, a secure airway, and need the trauma team at RGH.

When we arrive at RGH, Dr. Stein is waiting as we open the backdoors.

"What do have going on here, Mark?" he asked.

"We have Jeff and both of us are glad to see you," I said.

He nodded and said, "Okay, let's get Jeff into 12, he looks pretty sick."

Dr. Stein and I walked behind the team as they moved toward the main trauma room. I explained the scene and progression we've had along with a treatment summary.

Dr. Stein placed a chest tube into Jeff's right lateral chest. Blood flowed from the tube indicating heavy bleeding from the chest. Jeff was taken to the OR. He was later admitted to the trauma ICU.

He has a fractured sternum, three rib fractures, and pulmonary contusions. He had lost nearly half of his circulating blood volume by the time he arrived to the ED. He has fractures to most of the bones in the right side of his face and fractured skull.

We would follow Jeff's progress, and he remained in critical condition for several days before they had him stabilized and confident he would survive. It was an amazing survival story from as close to death as you could be.

We later learned his wife ended the backyard mechanics projects.

The next shift, after finishing the morning checks and washing rigs, we had scheduled training with Dennis who's our resident (hazardous materials) hazmat expert.

This is a required annual refresher class. Dennis is a volunteer EMT and part of the hazmat team. We're attending the training while on duty so the hope is to get it completed before the calls start.

We try to forget last year's class when we got called in the middle of the training for a disoriented female. When we arrived, the patient's daughter met us and explained her mother was acting strangely and couldn't get out of bed.

We entered the house and were immediately met with an overpowering fog of what smelled like ammonia and bleach. With eyes watering and occasional cough, we made it to the bedroom where the patient was unresponsive.

We learned the patient mixed ammonia and bleach while cleaning the bathroom to "get things cleaner" and it was nearly the demise of all of us.

After the transport, we agreed we wouldn't share the story with Dennis in fear of having to do the class a second time. The patient did fine and had a very clean but nearly lethal house.

We finished the training without interruption and, as always, learned some new things and hopefully would never have to use it. As we left the training room, the tones directed us to the rigs.

"Rescue 41, Medic 42, respond code three for an electrical worker on fire, at the Main Transformer Station, 1200 Douglas Street, time out 1254 hours."

Both crews made quick steps to the rigs and out the bay doors in less than twenty seconds. This sounded ominous and time could be a critical factor in determining the outcome.

Crew safety would be and is always paramount. When you're working around the electrical hazards associated with main transformers, there are no second chances. We would be following the lead of the experts on scene.

There's a flurry of activity going on as expected. We notice a worker in a yellow hard hat waving at us by a gated road. As we approach him, he's walking toward my window with a worried look about him.

"Down this road about fifty yards, he's hurt real bad," he said.

"Okay," I said and Rocky had us headed that direction.

Approaching the site, we find several workers kneeling in a semicircle around the patient who's sitting on the ground.

My first thought is, *He's alive.*

We're in the heart of the electrical transfer station, surrounded by a tall fence with menacing barbed razor wire; it has a look that says "Stay Out, Not Kidding!"

The structures around us are humming like a thousand angry bees, huge wires, and huge boxes; you can almost feel the energy, not a place I feel at ease being in.

We're informed today was a scheduled maintenance for one of the transformers. The patient was working next to it with a large wrench when somehow it made contact with something it shouldn't have, creating a spectacular arcing flash that engulfed our patient in a momentary hell.

This resulted in serious burns to his face and upper chest.

It then secondarily caught him on fire adding to the burns. He fortunately never received an electrical shock or lost consciousness. The coworkers were able to extinguish the fire using jackets and a dry chemical fire extinguisher.

He has most of his hair burned off, eyebrows are gone, the face has large blisters full of water and sagging, pieces of skin are hanging from his neck, lips are blistered and swollen, and there's heavy soot around his mouth.

His shirt is mostly burned off with pieces embedded in the skin and wisps of smoke from a piece near the collar.

This is a horrific and worst-case scenario; he most certainly has airway involvement, and on a proverbial clock, ticking down with not much time left in his favor.

I then hear a high-pitched and partially obstructed airway as he's moaning with pain.

This is stridor, the sound you never want to hear; the extreme swelling in the area of the epiglottis, down near the opening to the trachea, an area with not a lot of room for swelling.

We could literally have seconds before this guy loses his airway. Our immediate actions will determine if he lives or dies.

Rocky spoke up and said, "I'll get everything ready."

I knelt down to the patient and quickly introduced myself, "My name is Mark, I'm a paramedic, we're going to take care of you, and can you tell me your name?"

"Carl," he said in a forced, high-pitched response.

"Okay, Carl, just let us do our stuff. We're going to help you breathe and get you to the hospital," I told him and gently squeezed the top of his left shoulder.

He nodded very slowly. I cannot imagine the fear going through his mind.

Sam provided an oxygen mask over his mouth and nose, while Steve quickly began cutting the rest of his clothing.

I placed a rubber tourniquet on the right arm and called for a 14 gauge which Rocky handed me.

"Let's get set for the RSI," I said as I was taping the IV.

Dana finished drawing up the RSI drugs, and I made sure we were all on the same page. This would be vital to having a successful outcome on this no-room-for-error procedure.

Rocky had the laryngoscope, additional blades, the endotracheal tube, the suction, the bag valve mask all set out, and we're ready.

We gently laid Carl flat, and I looked at him making sure we made eye contact and said, "Here we go, Carl, hang on."

He just blinked once and stared back.

I pushed the etomidate which quickly rendered him unconscious. No turning back now.

Then the sux which induced paralysis and he stopped breathing. A couple of expected twitches and now it was up to me, there's no plan B, no other options, this has to work.

With the laryngoscope handle in my left hand, I gently inserted the blade into his mouth. From the onset, everything I see is red and swollen. There are pieces of soot all the way to the back of the throat. I found the epiglottis and suddenly have the smallest view of the vocal cords between the engorged tissues.

When you hear the stridorous sound a patient makes, it's unsettling, when you actually see the cause of it, it's frightening.

"Hand me the tube please," I said to Sam, without taking my eyes off the back of Carl's throat.

This tube would be smaller than one we would use if Carl's airway wasn't swelling. At this point, he needs the airway secured and this will accomplish that.

Sliding the tube down Carl's throat seemed like slow motion and then relief as I saw it pass through the vocal cords.

I closed my eyes for a second and said, "Let's get this secured and get moving."

Dana listened over Carl's chest with the stethoscope and held thumbs up indicating good air movement with each squeeze of the bag valve.

Rocky placed a large burn sheet on the gurney. We covered Carl with a second burn sheet and loaded him into the ambulance.

The burn sheets are about the size of a twin bed sheet. They are a sterile sheet to try to keep the burned areas as clean as possible in the prehospital setting.

It would take us seven minutes to reach RGH. In that time, we would notify them to have the trauma team standing by and still had a lot of work to do during the transport.

Burn injuries can be tremendously painful, even in Carl's unconscious state he could still be suffering.

I'm having Dana give incremental doses of morphine as long as the blood pressure remained stable. The goal was to give 20 mg before we reached RGH. This is a large but merciful start.

Sam was in charge of ventilations and focused all her attention to ensuring Carl was oxygenated and the endotracheal tube stayed in place. If it became dislodged at this point, we wouldn't be able to get it reinserted.

I found a couple areas on the chest I was able to attach the EKG electrodes and now had a view of the heart and vitals.

His EKG rhythm looks good. A little fast at 118 beats but that could be secondary to a pain response.

Blood pressure is 136/84 and the SpO2 is 96%.

We're not looking too bad here, I thought.

We arrived at RGH to a wonderful reception to get us into suite 12. Carl has an army of RGH's best taking care of him at this moment along with members of the burn unit.

After initial examination, they are estimating 36 percent third-degree burns or full-thickness and smaller percentages of various partial-thickness burns. The next few weeks will be Carl's critical period and much of that will be spent intubated and sedated.

We learned that Carl has worked for the county utilities department for the last seven years. He's married with a six-year-old son. Carl's life has changed forever, yet he's still the same guy and will go home to his family and that's what matters most of all.

Critical patients can present challenges at every aspect while in your care. This doesn't even take into consideration the emotional part of it. At the time of the treatment, there isn't time to reflect on much more than what needs to be done.

After the transport is completed, the call runs through your mind like a movie being played spitefully out of sequence.

"Did we do everything we could of?"

"Could we have done anything different?"

"Did we make a difference?"

Several shifts have gone by, and we are following Carl's progress. He's awake and still in the burn unit. His treatments are painful and agonizing but each day he's closer to his goal of going home.

EMS is a challenge. There are very few that would trade their experiences. Each call makes you stronger with your skills. No matter how long you're responding to calls for help, you can never know it all.

If you keep your eyes and ears open, you can learn something every shift.

15

TOO MUCH OR NOT ENOUGH

CERTAIN TIMES OF the year we tend to see increases in mental health-related emergencies. Holidays can be included on this list and certainly not everyone's a fan of the rainy season with dark and gloomy days. So with the upcoming festivities and forecast of bad weather over the next month, it isn't a good combination for EMS.

Dealing with psychiatric emergencies can be challenging. Any patient has the potential to act out aggressively, whether you are suffering with a mental or physical problem; you're not always in a rational frame of mind.

Today is a treat with heavy rains creating small lakes in places there shouldn't be and streets flooded as drains have trouble keeping up.

After getting the vehicle checks completed, we stood in front of the ambulance bay door watching one of these squalls coming down, creating a small torrent of water rushing down the street.

For some reason, it's fascinating watching small items being carried with the current: soda cans, sticks, a small box, and a trash can lid floating like a survival raft in choppy waters.

Dana is mesmerized by this with her hands above the glass on the big bay door and face almost touching the pane.

She resembles a cat standing tall over the back of the couch, staring out the window at a bird hopping across the lawn with tantalizing intent.

"Going to be fun going out in this stuff," Steve spoke up, interrupting the moment.

We didn't have to wait long to see if this would be true hearing the tones resonate through the bays.

"Rescue 41, Medic 42, respond code three for an attempted suicide by overdose, 111 Theodore Lane, time out 0848 hours."

Responding in this weather can delay our response. It doesn't do a patient any good if we don't show up because we were involved in a traffic collision. Driving with lights and siren is dangerous in sunny and dry conditions. Now add the rain and decreased visibility and the danger factor just went up exponentially.

We pulled up in front of the house and parked behind two police cars. We couldn't know if the patient was violent or maybe had unsecured weapons, issues far above our pay grade. We appreciate the safety the officers provide and always take comfort in seeing them here.

The front door opened as we approached it and an officer stepped out onto the porch.

"Hi guys, you have a nineteen-year-old male. We found several empty pill bottles. He scratched the labels off and doesn't recall the names or how many were in each bottle. He also has a four-page note describing how bad things are and how he wants his life to be over. He called 9-1-1 because he doesn't want to die at home...he wants to die in the hospital," he explained.

"Okay, we can check him out and see how we can help," I said.

"His name is Brad," the officer added.

With this information, we proceeded into the house.

Brad is lying on the couch and the other officer is standing next to him.

He's wearing jeans, no shoes or socks, and an ironic T-shirt with a large yellow smiley face that has a bullet hole to the head and blood dripping. The home is clean and obviously well taken care of.

I knelt down in front of the couch and kept space between us, "Brad, my name is Mark, I'm a paramedic. Can you tell me what's going on here today?" I asked.

It's important to respect the imaginary personal space that exists between people, especially when you're interviewing a patient that might not be in the mood for someone six inches in front of his face. It's also a safety factor, always be aware of your surroundings and have an escape route planned before you need it.

"Well, I want to die so I took a bunch of pills," he said without making eye contact.

"How long ago did you take these?" I asked.

"A long time ago," he said quietly staring away.

"Well, we need to take you to the hospital. Do you think you can make it onto the gurney?" I asked.

"I suppose," he said.

We got Brad into the ambulance and headed to RGH. Sam and Dana came since we didn't know what he'd taken or have any idea if he would *suddenly crash* and need resuscitated.

Dana was getting the LifePak 12 hooked up when Brad complained of being sleepy.

"You can sleep if you need to. We're just going to keep an eye on your heart. I also need to start an IV. Do you understand me?" I explained.

"Sure, as long as you give me something that speeds this process up, I thought the pills would have worked by now," he said.

"Well, I don't think I can help you with that one," I said.

After attaching the rubber tourniquet and finding a good vein, the IV went in. I inserted a plastic plug into the back of it which keeps the IV in a ready state.

We use this when we don't have a need for an IV bag hanging and slowly dripping fluids in.

The last step will include flushing a small amount of saline into the plug given through a syringe.

"Okay, Brad, the IV is in, I'm going to flush it with saline, you may feel a bit of cool liquid going up your arm," I said.

With a notable change in his demeanor, he looked down at the saline syringe going into the plastic plug and went absolutely ballistic.

He started fighting like a caged animal. Sam was trying to hold him from getting up without much success. Dana was literally lying across his legs, and I'm trying to duck and dodge the flailing punches wildly being thrown at anything and everywhere.

One of the last places on the planet you want to get into a knock-down, drag-out death match is in the back of an ambulance.

Brad is screaming at the top of his lungs, "I don't want to die, I don't want to die, don't inject me, don't inject me."

Brad is maybe 160 pounds, not too muscular. He has the advantage going at 100 percent while we're trying to get him under control without causing injury.

Rocky pulled the ambulance over and quickly came to help us. Steve was following in the rescue but little he could do as there was no more room.

It took the four of us several minutes before we had him positioned on his stomach with seat belts securing him from moving.

During the struggle, his IV was ripped out along with the EKG patches from the LifePak 12.

The first two buttons on Sam's shirt were ripped off, Dana was kicked in the face, and Rocky and I were panting as if we ran up five flights of stairs.

Brad continued to struggle under the straps. His efforts were less intense and didn't respond to any questions or commands we directed to him.

I made the decision to hold on giving him an antipsychotic medication on the potential it would act with whatever medication he'd taken.

We radioed ahead to RGH to have security standing by.

There were four guards to meet us. We went to suite 9 where Brad was transferred from our gurney to the ED gurney and restrained with soft restraints.

We're fortunate no one was injured during this episode other than Dana's fat lip. It's a stark reminder of the potential hostilities we can face at any given time on any given day. You can never let your guard down or become complacent.

Brad had elevated levels of acetylsalicylic acid (aspirin) in his system.

It's unlikely this triggered his violent outburst. In his chart, he was diagnosed as having bipolar disorder with violent episodes. He was admitted to the psychiatric floor and expected to make a full recovery.

Back at the station, things were pretty much back to normal. Dana had the only visible injury, a swollen lip she was nursing with a bag of frozen corn.

After lunch, the rains let up and it was now just sprinkling. The skies were dark and ominous looking like it could let loose with a downpour any minute. So far we'd been fortunate to not have any weather-related calls.

The rest was short-lived with the tones directing us to the bays.

"Rescue 41, Medic 42, respond code three for a male in his sixties with chest pain, 5420 Barlow Drive, time out 1414 hours."

We made it out the station and found traffic quite light. Maybe the weather had something to do with it; everyone was hunkered down at home. Good place for them.

This address would take five minutes to get to. After a couple of minutes, we got an update from dispatch.

"Rescue 41, Medic 42, be advised your patient just lost consciousness, he is on the floor, and we are attempting to get more information, the wife has disconnected the line."

Steve and I both received the update. We'll be on scene in less than one minute.

The front door of the residence was open. As we exited the vehicles, the wife came to the door pleading for us to, "Please hurry."

We find the patient supine (face up) on the living room floor.

He's ghostly pale and a small pile of vomit a few feet away from his head. His eyes are open, but he doesn't respond to my initial greeting to him.

"Ma'am, can you tell us what happened here?" I asked.

"He was having pains in his chest. He took one of his pills and after I called you he got sick and fainted," she explained.

I gave him some more of his pills and that's it," she said.

"Can you show me the pills?" I said.

She left and went into the other room.

Sam cut his shirt open and hooked up the LifePak 12.

The first heart rate is 30 beats per minute. The blood pressure will not read.

He has no radial pulses and his carotid pulse is weak and slow. His breathing is shallow about twelve per minute.

His wife returns and hands me an empty bottle of nitroglycerin tablets.

"How many did you give him?" I asked, starting to have a bad feeling about this.

"Well, I don't know, they're so small, I put some of them under his tongue," she said.

I looked into his mouth with a penlight and see several small little white nitro pills under his tongue and scattered throughout his mouth.

Nitroglycerin tablets are for patients with known coronary artery disease, specifically angina pectoris.

Angina pectoris is a form of heart disease. It's a progressive narrowing of the coronary arteries which are the arteries that provide the heart muscle itself with blood. During exertion or spontaneously, the heart muscle can become starved for oxygen and the patient will have sharp, squeezing, burning, dull, or crushing chest pain.

One pill is then placed under the tongue and dissolved slowly. Its effects are to increase the size of the coronary artery and thus deliver more oxygen to the heart muscle and theoretically reduce the chest pain.

You cannot take more than one pill every five minutes and then generally a maximum of three.

The nitro tablets can have a secondary effect of lowering the overall blood pressure and due caution must be used when taking them. He now has enough pills in his mouth to lower his blood pressure to zero, causing death.

I looked at Rocky and Steve and with urgency said, "We need to get these out his mouth, now."

We rolled the patient onto his side and have to be careful about sticking fingers into his mouth. (We want to keep all ten of them just the way they are.) I continued to use the penlight and managed to get twelve of the pills out and couldn't see any others.

Sam has an oxygen mask over his mouth and nose, and Dana has an IV bag set and ready.

As I look at the LifePak 12 it's now showing a heart rate of 24.

I still feel a slow, faint carotid pulse.

We have to start pacing his heart which will hopefully keep him from going in to cardiac arrest.

We'll place the large combo pads on his chest which are used for delivering shocks. The LifePak 12 will deliver small amounts of electricity which will stimulate the heart and generate a higher pulse rate than 24.

I'm setting the pacer to 80 beats per minute. When it's switched on, the patient's chest immediately begins twitching 80 times a minute as the electricity is being delivered.

It's not particularly painful, some patient's report intolerance and others tolerance.

We now need the IV in for fluids.

With his blood pressure so low, he needs fluid infused to raise the pressure until the effects of the nitro wear off which could be up to another fifteen minutes or more.

He has an empty tank.

After getting the rubber tourniquet on the right arm, I found a good vein to get a 16 gauge into. We're now pouring the fluid in rapidly. We still have no blood pressure reading.

I carry more powerful medications that can reduce the size of his blood vessels. I will administer this if things don't improve very quickly.

After nearly emptying the entire bag of fluid, Dana calls out the latest numbers, pacer at 80, blood pressure 66/32, and SpO2 won't read," she said.

We're heading the right direction. Sam has a second IV bag ready, and I am searching for sites. I notice a small vein in the back of the left hand. I get a 20 gauge into it and now have both IV bags flowing wide open.

We're still not getting any verbal response from the patient. Dana calls out the next blood pressure reading, "74/44."

I think we may have turned him around.

Time to get him lifted to the gurney and headed to RGH.

A look at the front door, it's absolutely pouring. We need to construct a cover in order to keep the patient dry. We're not worried about the electricity being delivered in the rain but we don't want him soaked and have the EKG patches or any of the tape from the IVs coming loose.

Rocky has a sheet from the ambulance, and Dana, Sam, Steve, and Rocky all have a corner, and we are slowly moving to the ambulance while holding this tarp over the patient. It worked well other than we all got soaked.

With both IV bags flowing, we now have a blood pressure reading of 80/50.

The patient does look at me as I call his name and is following simple commands, like "squeeze my fingers."

His grips are equal on both sides. We're continuing the pacing at 80 beats per minute.

We had the cardiac team standing by and taking over care in suite 4. They're going to turn the pacer off and prepared to reinstitute it if needed.

As they turn it off, the heart rate drops to 30, and they immediately start pacing again. He's headed to the cath lab to have an internal pacemaker inserted, a permanent one.

Our patient's name is Max. He's sixty-eight years old and worked on the railroad for forty-five years. We can only imagine there'll be some spousal education about the use of nitro.

We're going back to the station to dry out, for now.

Rocky got off the phone with Rachel. She's finishing her shift at the ED and wanted us to know Max had a pacemaker inserted and stabilized in the CCU. She said he was awake and didn't remember the transport into the hospital.

He was very fortunate as he could have had a worse outcome.

The rains have let up for the last few hours and now it's just cloudy and cool. Good weather to stay inside and be warm. We couldn't be that fortunate as the tones had us heading to the bays.

"Rescue 41, Medic 42, respond code three to the county jail for an unconscious male, enter off the south wing, time out 2055 hours."

We occasionally respond to the jail for everything from sick people to assaults, to attempted suicides. We provide the same high level of care regardless who our patient is. It can be challenging as the inmates are not beyond plotting for either getting pain medications or even planning escapes.

Medics have also been assaulted. We'll be vigilant and watch each other's back.

After a four-minute response we're in front of the secure roll-up door on the south wing. The door slowly raises and we drive into the structure. Steve, Sam, and Dana will leave the rescue parked outside.

As we park inside the large garage, the door closes behind us. Rocky pulled the gurney and the equipment is loaded onto it, and we're awaiting the elevator which will take us to the second floor. The elevator has no buttons; it's controlled by a main control room via closed-circuit monitoring.

This procedure is part of a built-in safety precaution that prevents escapes.

As we arrive on the second floor, two correctional officers are there to direct us to the patient. They will also remain with us throughout the visit.

"Hi guys, we got a kid who's unresponsive. He's been acting odd since he got here an hour ago and now he's just kind of lying there. He came to us after a burglary arrest. He's been keeping to himself and that's about all we know. He denied any medical history or suicidal ideations," the officer informed us.

"Okay, we can give him the once-over and see if we can figure out what's going on with him," I said.

After walking through two additional locked doors, we're at the end of a block of cells. As the door opens to the cell in front of us, we see the patient lying in his bunk. His face is ashen color, and he's snoring about every third or fourth breath. He also looks to be drenched with sweat.

"Let's get him down to the floor guys. We need to figure out what's going on here. He's not looking too good," I said.

Steve and Rocky lifted him to the floor. He doesn't respond during this move. Sam's at the top of his head aligning his airway, and Dana has an oxygen mask over his mouth and nose.

"He's soaked," Dana said.

"Yeah, I noticed that, we better check his sugar level pretty quick, and make sure we're not missing an insulin shock cause," I said.

Insulin shock is a critically low blood sugar. It means the body has too much insulin and needs sugar. It can come on in several different ways. When someone takes their insulin, by an injection to the abdomen, they have to balance it out by eating something soon after the shot, maybe they missed a meal, or perhaps even took too much intentionally.

Rocky has the kit open and setting an IV up.

Suddenly, the kid starts grand mal seizing, and Dana quickly grabs a blanket and puts it under his head to protect him from the cement floor. The seizure lasts for forty-five seconds and now he's moaning and choking on secretions.

Sam is suctioning while Dana is holding the oxygen mask next to his mouth and nose.

I put the tourniquet on his right arm above the elbow. A good vein popped up in the back of the hand, which I prefer in case he seizes again. If I put the IV in the midarm, it could become compromised with the violent contractions.

The IV goes in and I'm using extra tape. We won't be losing this IV.

"Sugar says LO," Rocky called out.

That confirms it, we have insulin shock. With the LO reading, we know his sugar level is below 20, normal is 70–100.

Rocky hands me the dextrose, it's called D50. This is a large bolus of concentrated sugar water given through the IV line.

The patient response is usually quick; similar to Narcan with the narcotic overdose patient.

I have the D50 syringe in the IV port and begin pushing the plunger. Within seconds, the patient opens his eyes and looks around suspiciously.

"Hey there, can you hear me?" I asked.

"Uh-huh, where am I?" he asked with near-genuine confusion.

"We're in the jail, do you remember what happened?" I asked as I finished with the D50.

"Jail...how'd I get in here?" he asked, again with confusion.

"Are you a diabetic?" I asked.

"Yeah, but why am I in jail?" he asked again.

This was getting strange. His demeanor and question line are very convincing for at least *some* additional investigation.

"Do you use insulin?" I asked.

"Yeah, I do, I don't understand what's going on!" he said.

Sam was getting blood pressure readings, and Dana was rechecking the sugar as I went to talk to the officer.

"My recommendation is we take him to RGH where they can monitor him a little closer, and resolve if he's been out of it or what's going on here," I said.

"Sure, okay, sounds good, this is odd," the officer said.

The patients name is James; he's twenty-six years old. We would learn he's never had so much as a parking ticket. He was found wandering in a business near his home. There were no signs of forced entry, the door was apparently open and he walked in.

"Sugar is 166," Dana called out.

"Roger that, thanks, Dana," I said.

After we give the D50, the sugar level comes up rapidly. He will need to eat a more solid meal at RGH as the bolus we just administered will not sustain him very long.

The transport to RGH was uneventful. James continued to try to piece together where his last few hours went.

Between the physicians at RGH and detectives, they determined he was in insulin shock and unaware of being in the store or having the intent to burglarize it.

He was released and ordered to follow up with his primary care physician to evaluate his current insulin regimen.

16

DISPATCH...
WE'VE BEEN HIT!

ON THE WEEKENDS, the crew have the station to themselves. Rachel has the day off and came to visit Rocky. Of course, the kids have to come along, and they're always the life of the station.

Hank goes straight to the kitchen and makes sure we've done a good job cleaning and not left anything too close to the counter needing his further inspection. Abby is happiest with whoever gives the most attention and then kisses are freely dispensed. Kelsey keeps an eye on Hank and Abby and goes to where the most action is at the time.

At the public entrance to the station, the door is locked on the weekends and after hours during the week. There's a bell that rings in the crew quarters and a public phone that's a direct line to dispatch for citizens that might drive up needing assistance.

Everyone's in the day room thoroughly entertained by Hank and Abby having a tug-of-war with a rope while Kelsey is randomly playfully biting their necks.

Suddenly the front entrance bell rings several times in succession.

Steve and I head that way and can see a man looking through the window and then waving as he sees Steve and me coming toward him.

We open the door and he quickly says, "I have my mother-in-law in the car, we think she may have had a stroke and she broke her foot."

"Steve, I'll go out and have a look, call dispatch and let them know what we're doing, and Rocky, bring the ambulance around," I said.

"Roger that," Steve said and Rocky headed to the bay.

There's a four-door sedan parked in the front lot. The back passenger side door is open where an elderly female is sitting, staring ahead, and doesn't look to be in distress.

A younger female is standing next to the open door with a worried look.

As I walked toward the car, the man is walking with me and explaining, "We went to check on her because she wasn't answering the phone. We found her in the yard walking in circles near the back of the property. She can't speak and her foot is nearly broke off," he said.

The female standing outside the car steps aside and says, "This is my mother Anita, she needs help."

"Okay, we'll do the best we can," I said and knelt down next to Anita.

The first thing I notice is Anita's right foot; it's a terrifying presentation, bent over just hanging there, attached by the smallest of tissues.

To my surprise and horror, she tried to get out of the seat when I knelt down and *lifted* the right leg as if to get out of the car. When she did, the foot swung wildly as if attached to a string.

I quickly stopped her from moving any further by placing my right hand below her right knee and left hand on her right shoulder.

"Please don't move, Anita. I'm going to help you, I need you to stay still," I said.

I then noticed a slight left facial droop and didn't see any movement on her left side.

I looked back at her daughter and asked, "Is this facial droop and weakness on her left side new?"

"Yes, she was fine last night when I spoke to her," she said in between sobs.

Sam and Dana walked up as Rocky was pulling up in the ambulance.

While still holding the right leg from moving, I explained what we had to Sam and Dana.

Dana quickly got into the back of the ambulance. She used a cardboard splint, cut and shaped it into a half boot. This fit perfectly to the right lower leg and after a couple wraps of tape we're ready to lift Anita onto the stretcher.

Steve has the daughter and son-in-law off to the side explaining what was going to happen and where we'd be taking her.

We can only surmise Anita had a stroke sometime today. She then went outside and at some point fractured the right ankle. She kept walking on it, nearly completely amputating it by the time she was discovered.

It's not uncommon for a stroke patient to have an altered mental status. It can create a dangerous situation as evidenced today by Anita.

In the back of the ambulance we're able to get a better assessment of her condition. She cannot speak and any attempt is garbled and unintelligible. She has no coordinated movement on the left side.

Sam has Anita on oxygen by mask. She's also talking to her explaining what we're doing. Even though Anita cannot speak or acknowledge us, we believe she can understand everything and can only imagine she's terrified.

I'm trying to find an IV site while Dana got the LifePak 12 hooked up and calling numbers for me.

"Heart rate 60, blood pressure 240/140, and SpO2 98%," she said.

The blood pressure prompted a double-take at the EKG screen. Anita is having a significant neurological event, and we need to get her to the neurosurgeons at RGH, and quickly.

I found a site for an IV and after getting it secured checked her sugar level.

"110 on the sugar," Dana said looking down at the glucometer screen.

"Roger that, 110," I said.

I decided to give Anita increments of morphine which would do two things: First, it would help with any pain she was potentially having from the ankle, and secondly, it could have a calming effect and perhaps lower the blood pressure.

By the time we arrived at RGH, I'd given 10 mg of morphine.

Anita was slightly more relaxed and blood pressure had come down to 216/126, still critical.

Anita suffered a major stroke. At seventy-six years old, her only history was high blood pressure. She's admitted to the ICU, and after stabilization, going to the OR to attempt to save her right foot.

The prognosis would be guarded. With physical therapy, it's possible to regain some of the lost movement.

The station was empty when we got back, Rachel and the kids had gone home. We're now in the discussion mode for what everyone wants to do about dinner.

"Pizza," Dana called out.

"I second that," Sam concurred.

Rocky opened his mouth to respond but was covered by tones reverberating through the station.

"Rescue 41, Medic 42, respond code three for a twenty-eight-year-old female, she is unconscious and in seizure, 506 Bryant Street, time out 1648 hours."

For a weekend, traffic is very light. We'll be on scene in less than four minutes. Seizures can occur for many reasons; some of which can be life threatening. Getting to the scene quickly could make a difference.

Pulling up to the residence, we see a male in his twenties. He's standing in the doorway of the residence and waving.

As we walk up, he says, "She's still having the seizure, follow me."

We're led into a large room where another male is kneeling on the floor cradling the female patient while she's having an active grand mal seizure.

A grand mal seizure involves nearly every muscle in the body convulsing at the same time. They're usually self-limiting but can last several minutes. This seizure has been going on for two minutes.

Her husband is the one cradling her. He explained what happened.

"Thirty minutes ago, Chrissie had a sudden headache and had to lie down on the couch in the office. I came into check on her and couldn't wake her up, and then she started to have this seizure. She runs five miles every day and is the picture of health," he said.

Sam is placing an oxygen mask over Chrissie's mouth and nose. After another thirty seconds, the seizure has stopped. She's become a terrible color of purple across her face and fingernails. This is from hypoxia, lack of oxygen.

Chrissie is now having *posturing* in which her arms and legs are abnormally extending in a rigid posture. This is an ominous sign.

With the history of the sudden headache and subsequent seizure, Chrissie could have a cerebral hemorrhage or brain bleed which can potentially be catastrophic.

Dana has the LifePak 12 hooked up and the numbers I am hearing are frightening.

"Heart rate 50, blood pressure 180/130, and SpO2 at 85%," Dana called out.

We need to expedite the transport and continue treatment on the way. I'm going to get an IV in while Rocky and Steve are getting Chrissie loaded onto the gurney. This will be our lifeline for the RSI procedure and any other drugs we need to administer.

I quickly met with Chrissie's husband and friend.

"My name is Mark, I'm a paramedic, we'll be taking Chrissie to Regional, we'll get her there quickly, and they'll continue helping her there," I explained.

"Is she going to be okay?" her husband asked, almost as if he sensed this was every bit as serious as it looked.

"Well, she's very sick, the important part is getting her to Regional," I said.

"Okay, we'll meet you there, please tell her I love her," he said.

I nodded and walked out to the ambulance.

Rocky has us headed to RGH with lights and siren activated. I have the drugs drawn up for the RSI. Chrissie responds quickly becoming flaccid and stopped breathing as planned.

With the laryngoscope in hand, I quickly find the vocal cords and the intubation goes without difficulty.

Dana has the bag valve and watching Chrissie's chest rise and fall with each squeeze of the bag.

During the reassessment, Chrissie's right pupil is blown and nonreactive. This is a dilated pupil and generally secondary to rising intracranial pressure, another worrying sign.

She's in fit, excellent-looking health as her husband described. I notice her wedding ring and perfectly manicured fingernails. Her appearance does not reflect the massive insult her brain is suffering.

Dana is next to Chrissie's ear telling her what we're doing. I then shared Chrissie's husband's request to Dana and she immediately went back to her left ear.

You can't teach what Sam, Dana, Steve, and Rocky bring to every scene we go to. Dana is treating Chrissie, not just a patient.

We arrived and went straight to suite 12. Chrissie was quickly taken to CT scan and the news is devastating. She has a massive subarachnoid bleed and is being prepped for emergency brain surgery.

Chrissie died on the OR table at 1805 hours.

Over the next few shifts, we've been a BLS medic unit, Basic Life Support. Not that this is a bad thing; in fact it's a good thing. This means our calls are non-life-threatening and very benign. Of course, the person being transported wouldn't call it benign.

When you crash your bicycle on a leisurely ride and fracture your wrist, and you're three miles from home, and have to have a passerby call 9-1-1, and your dog is home waiting for you to get back so they can do their business, it certainly isn't benign to them.

Coming on duty this morning it's a miracle any of us made it to the station. The rains are causing flooding, car crashes, power outages, and making travel hazardous. We're finishing our morning routines of vehicle and equipment checks.

"Man, listen to that rain. Can our little station here take much more?" Rocky exclaimed.

"Do you really mean the station or are you actually talking about yourself?" I asked.

"Let's just hurry up and get done so we can watch stuff float down the street," Dana intervened.

"Any bets on the first call?" Steve asked.

"Well you know—" and Rocky was interrupted by the tones not allowing any guessing as they echoed throughout the bay.

"Rescue 41, Medic 42, Engine 61, respond code three for a vehicle rollover on State Highway 4, Milepost 6, we're getting multiple calls on this, time out 0855 hours."

Another area we share with District 6. This will be a welcome response as their engine provides great protection on scenes where you're working around traffic.

Both units went en route, and we're driving with due caution secondary to not being able to see more than a couple of car lengths ahead. Traffic is light, and we have that to our advantage.

Someone's out in this because we're going to their rollover.

State Highway 4 is a 65 mph three-lane freeway. The area we're responding to has a couple of curves that require attention but driven defensively they're no problem. There are moderate embankments on this stretch and sounds like the car stayed on the road which makes the extrication easier.

We're arriving and there's a midsized car on its top in lane number one, the far right lane. There are several cars pulled over and a couple people standing next to the driver's door leaning over and looking in the vehicle.

Rocky pulls the ambulance ahead of the rollover, and Steve's parking the Rescue a car length behind which gives us some protection as we're assessing and extricating the patient.

The rain is relentless.

Traffic is moving past us at freeway speeds in lanes two and three. It's unsettling as the wind and spray is felt as each car passes.

Sam went to the passenger side of the car. The window is broken so she crawls through easily and at the patient's side.

The driver is the sole occupant.

Engine 61 has arrived and parked a couple car lengths behind Rescue 41 and partially in lane number one.

I'm able to talk to the patient from the driver's window.

"Hello there, can you hear me? My name is Mark, I'm a paramedic, we're here to help you," I called out.

"Yeah, what happened?" the elderly patient is asking slowly.

"Well, it looks like you rolled your car, are you hurt anywhere?"

"My right shoulder is sore, and my knee," he said.

"Okay, what is your name, sir?"

"Wilson, just call me Wilson."

"Okay, Wilson, we're going to get you out of there and take you to Regional, and get you checked out, sounds like a plan?" I asked.

"Okay, good luck, we may need a boat, it's raining pretty heavy."

"Well, I think we'll be okay for now."

Rocky is preparing equipment in the ambulance and suspiciously staying dry. Steve has the backboard, and Dana is standing next to him.

"Mark, he's free from everything. If you send the board in through the window, I can get him secured," Sam called out from inside the car.

"Okay, Sam, sounds like a plan," I agreed.

Steve sent the board through the open window, foot end first and between Sam and I, we have Wilson secure.

"Okay, Steve, we can start pulling him out, slowly," I said.

Two of the firefighters from Engine 61 are holding a tarp over our small working area and shielding us from some of the rain. They'll continue this over Wilson as we get him onto the gurney and into the ambulance.

We have Wilson out, and Sam is inching her way back out the passenger side of the car.

Sam stood up to brush her pants off when a scream of alert coming from Capt. Neeves was heard. The last thing I saw was Sam going flying, like a rag doll, over the embankment.

"Watch out, he's gonna hit us!" was the imminent warning.

Then the sickening sounds of the crash, everything going dark, and strange silence, I'm then aware of rain falling on my face.

A car traveling at over 60 mph hydroplaned and lost control, Capt. Neeves saw it heading toward us and yelled out.

Rescue 41 was violently slammed into Wilson's vehicle just behind the driver's door, missing Wilson and me by mere inches.

The two District 6 firefighters jumped back and were clear, they're shaken but okay.

Steve is lying next to Dana and they're both on their backs, okay and slowly getting up.

Steve and I looked at each other, and I said, "Steve, call dispatch, send help, Sam's down!"

"Dispatch, this is Rescue 41, we've been hit by another vehicle, repeat we've been hit, send a second ambulance and Rescue to our location, we have a crew member down," was Steve's broadcast.

Steve's voice was deliberate. The tone reflective of the ultimate professional he is. Dispatch immediately acknowledged the transmission; you could hear their concern as well.

One of the District 6 firefighters looked at me and said, "We got Wilson, go to Sam."

Steve and I were quickly on the other side of the overturned vehicle and looking over the embankment. It's fifteen feet to the bottom, and Sam is lying face down, not moving.

Rocky and Dana have the kit and another long spine board; we're stunned, numb with fear not knowing if Sam was dead or alive.

I walked a few steps forward as to not rain dirt and rocks down on her and quickly made my way down the embankment. Steve is right behind me.

As I make it to Sam, I hear the most wonderful sound; first she moaned, then her breathing.

I have my hands on both sides of her head to prevent her from moving and got next to her ear.

"Hey you, can you hear me? Can you talk to me?" I asked.

"Aah…Aah, what just happened?" she asked in a sleepy, fuzzy sounding voice.

"We got hit, Sam, do you hurt anywhere?"

"My hip, my left hip, I think that's it," she said, starting to sound more alert.

"Okay, don't move, you know the drill, we're taking you to Regional."

Back at the top of the hill, I saw Holly Ryan, a paramedic from District 3; she has the most terrified look on her face.

I looked at her with the biggest smile and nodded affirmatively.

She waved with a relieved grin and pointed at Wilson making an "okay" sign with her right hand.

Sam has a radial pulse of 110; she's alert, breathing okay, and I don't find any other injuries.

We have her secured to the spine board and getting ready to climb the hill.

I notice she's trying to get my attention. I bent over and place my left ear in front of her face.

"Mark, please don't RSI me, and no 14 gauge, and *don't* cut my clothes off," she whispered.

"Hmm, well, you're getting two of the three, you decide which one you don't need," I said and winked at her.

We made it to the top of the hill and to the gurney, and into the ambulance. Steve's remaining on scene with the Rescue, it will need towed.

The driver who lost control was uninjured and is sitting in a state patrol car getting multiple tickets.

We're headed to RGH and need to ensure Sam isn't injured and we aren't missing anything.

The first thing she's getting is clothes cut off. Dana left the small underclothes on.

She then hooked up the LifePak 12 and covered Sam with a blanket.

"Heart rate at 112, blood pressure at 106/60, and SpO2 at 97%," Dana called out.

"Roger that," I said.

"Did you know the lights are really dirty?" Sam said out of the blue.

Dana and I were startled by this until we noticed Sam staring at the ceiling.

"I heard that," Rocky called out from the front.

"What do you have bionic hearing?" Sam called out.

Sam was then surprised by the *tap-tap-tap* to her vein followed by the IV I put into her left midarm.

"Ouch, was that a 14?" she asked.

"Of course not, it was only a 16," I said.

Repeating the secondary assessment, I'm checking head to toe, there's ecchymosis (bluish discoloration) to the left hip just below the beltline, and I don't feel any crepitus (bone grinding) or instability. Her color is good, breath sounds are clear, no numbness or tingling, very fortunate to even be alive.

We arrived to RGH and half the ED is on hand to ensure Sam was well taken care of.

I went out to the ambulance where Rocky and Dana were cleaning.

"That's as close as I ever want to get. That could have taken all of us," I surmised.

"Can we go back to the station and disconnect everything?" Rocky asked.

"Trust me, I thought about it," I said.

Sam would stay at RGH for the next two hours, x-rays and monitoring. Nick is coming in to fill in on the Rescue for the rest of the shift.

Steve drove up in the spare Rescue, and the first words out his mouth are, "How is she?"

"She's fine, Steve, going to be her old self next shift," I said.

He smiled and went into the ED followed by Dana and Rocky. After several minutes, they came out and we're ready to head back to the station.

"I'll be right there guys," I yelled.

I went back to suite 12, and Sam was alone. They have her off the spine board and she's in a reclined position and smiles as I walk in.

"You kind of gave me a little scare out there I'll have you know," I said.

"I think it would take more than a car slamming into me at 60 mph," Sam said and held a thumb up.

I leaned over and gave her a hug and nod, and turned to walk out.

"Hey, thanks for not RSI'ing me," she said.

I walked back and rested both hands on the side rail of her bed and said, "No problem, Sam, and by the way, *purple*? And where did you get that *tan*?" I asked and then quickly moved toward the door.

"Oh you are so..." was all I heard before leaving the room.

17

ALEX'S DAY

THE EMS COUNCIL sponsored an EMT class in a neighboring department. The students had completed their final testing and were now looking for opportunities to complete their required ride time on the ambulance. As part of their class requirements, they'll spend up to three shifts and try to have some active role on at least five calls. This could be obtaining vital signs or any other procedure they would be performing in the duties of practicing as an EMT. They would also have the benefit of the safety net of the crew.

Today, we have Alex riding with us. He's twenty-one years old and a volunteer with District 6.

The morning started as it does every shift with completing vehicle checks and going over all the supplies and equipment. Alex was in the middle of it all and trying to take everything in.

"So you have it all down and ready to run the first call of the day?" I asked.

With a bewildered gaze and nervous expression, he replied, "Oh sure, no problem, piece of cake, no pressure or anything like that."

"Well, we all started right where you are, it'll come, have the faith," I said.

"Our instructor told us stories about you guys, and how if he was ever hurt or really sick, he would want the Station 4 crew," he said.

"Well, don't believe everything you hear, Alex," I said and held a thumbs up sign.

Sam walked around the corner, a slight limp but claiming to be 100 percent.

"Don't worry, Alex, we'll help you, right to the front of the call," she said with a pat to Alex's right shoulder that startled him.

And that conversation was stopped short by tones, and Alex's first call of the day toward becoming an EMT.

"Rescue 41, Medic 42, respond code three for a sixty-five-year-old female, not breathing, 4700 Pine Street, time out 0855 hours."

Alex stood in front of the passenger door before quickly turning around and nearly running into me, "Sorry, I meant to get in the other door," he said and then stepped into the side door and buckled up in the airway—jump seat.

We should be on scene within four minutes as traffic is light. Most of the morning rush-hour crowd is already off the streets.

"Rescue 41, Medic 42, we're getting reports the patient may have started breathing...the caller can't give us any more information."

Steve and I both acknowledged the update.

We arrived and quickly made it to the front door of the residence. After several seconds, a female came to the door with a distressed look.

"It's my mother, she's blue and won't wake up, hurry," she said and took off leading the way.

We followed her down a short hall and into a bedroom on the left. Her mother is lying in bed, as she described, unresponsive and blue.

Steve and Rocky were about to lift her to the floor when she opened her eyes and took two small breaths.

Rocky checked her carotid pulse announcing, "She has a strong pulse, feels like about 100."

Sam looked at Alex and motioned for him to help her with the bag valve mask.

"I'll do the squeezing, you get the seal over her face," Sam directed him.

This was brilliant on Sam's part, being able to manage an airway is the bread and butter of being an EMT. Alex will sink or swim after being thrown into the deep end of the proverbial pool by Sam.

With hands shaking, Alex positioned the mask over the patient's mouth and nose and nodded to Sam.

Sam squeezed the bag and fluttering sounds were heard as air went everywhere except into the mouth. He repositioned his hands, grabbed the jaw a little tighter and on the second try air went in and we all noticed the patient's chest rise.

"Good job, Alex," I said.

With a focused look and tense grin, he nodded slightly.

After a few more squeezes of the bag, the blue color started to be replaced by a more lifelike color.

Dana got the LifePak 12 hooked up.

"Heart rate 94, blood pressure 80/52, and SpO2 is 92%," she called out.

"Can you tell us what happened?" I asked her daughter.

"Well, she never sleeps this late. I came to check on her and she wouldn't wake up and she was blue, I thought she was dead," she said and started crying.

"Did she complain about anything or have any recent problems?" I asked.

"She had her knee scoped yesterday and came home last night but that's it. She took her pain pills and went to sleep," she explained.

That statement about the pain pills sparked my interest.

I bent over and opened the patient's eyes and found our problem; her pupils are pinpoint, she's overdosed on narcotics.

"Do you have the bottle of pain medication?" I asked her daughter.

"Yeah I'll go get it," she said and left the room.

She came back and said, "It's gone, I don't know where she put it."

Alex spoke up and said, "There's a bottle on the table, behind the tissues there."

Sure enough this was the missing bottle. It was a script of Vicodin for twenty pills, with twelve missing.

Either intentionally or accidental, she OD'd on narcotics.

I put an IV in the back of her left hand. We have everyone in position as I slowly pushed the Narcan through the IV line.

Within seconds, she opened her eyes and looked around the room.

"What are you doing here?" she asked.

"Mom, you took too many pills for Christ's sake, what were you thinking, you scared me half to death," her daughter exclaimed angrily.

"Did you take more than you should have?" I asked her.

"Well, I can't remember. My knee hurt and I took a few of them, there wasn't that many anyway," she admitted.

"Mom, you heard the pharmacist tell you to be careful with those, did you *not* listen to him?" she again said angrily.

"Okay...okay, I think we're doing better, let's just get to Regional and we can figure out the rest there," I said, trying to spare "Mom" any more verbal punishment.

We got her safely secured on the gurney and into the ambulance where Alex was the star. He was checking vital signs, readjusting her pillow; anything to make her more comfortable. We were just along for the ride.

After the transport and getting the ambulance back together, I asked Alex what he thought.

"I was pretty nervous," he said.

"I thought maybe we could ease into it with something simple but that was intense, nothing like practicing in class," he added.

I told him, "Well, you did a great job. Your first call as an EMT and your first save."

We made it back to the station and ate lunch uninterrupted. I had paperwork to catch up on, and Alex was getting training with the crew. When we have a new EMT, they get the full benefit, whether we have calls or not.

You can never go over the equipment *too much*. Sam, Dana, Steve, and Rocky have Alex in the training room, and I'm not sure if I should go rescue him or join in on the flow of information they're "injecting" into him.

We certainly don't expect he'll walk out here remembering half of it. But it gets stored up there somewhere in the old memory, and that knowledge might be triggered to guide him when he faces that critical moment on a critical patient.

After sixty minutes, Alex must have needed a break, and the EMS gods gave it to him with tones resonating throughout the station.

"Rescue 41, Medic 42, respond code three for an unknown medical problem, 1411 23rd Avenue, law enforcement also being advised, time out 1555 hours."

Alex closed the side door of the ambulance and once again got buckled into the airway seat.

"How'd the training go?" I asked.

"Wow, I thought EMT training was a lot, how'd you guys get to know all this stuff?" he asked.

"Just like you're doing, Alex, coming in here and riding and going on calls, we learn something new every day," I explained.

Alex was about to add more to that thought when dispatch interrupted with an update.

"Rescue 41, Medic 42, you have a sixteen-year-old female, she is reportedly out of control and possibly on mushrooms."

Steve and I both acknowledged the update.

Mushrooms are hallucinogenic and can result in loss of mind control with horrifying experiences for the user. They're illegal and can make treatment difficult as there's no antidote to reverse the effects. Also the patient can be irrational and unpredictable.

We're arriving in front of the residence and park behind two police cars.

After grabbing all the equipment, we can hear blood-curdling screams coming from inside and we're still at the curbside.

We walk into the house, one of the officers is standing in the kitchen facing the patient; she's on her hands and knees going in rapid circles while shaking her head violently and screaming.

Her hair is disheveled and completely covering her face. She has superficial scratches up and down both arms.

She's wearing underwear, one sock and a sports bra.

There's a second young female and young male seated on the couch in the living room; the other officer is standing in front of them with his notepad.

He comes over to us and explained, "Hi guys, apparently they all ate mushrooms an hour ago, and your patient started getting out of control shortly thereafter. She's cut herself with a kitchen knife, and now we can't seem to get anything out of her. Her name is Deena," he said.

"Okay, well, we need to try to get her secured and go from there," I explained.

This will not be an easy approach and it will be impossible to judge how she will react.

"Dana, you want to see if you can get her to respond to you," I said.

Dana looked at me like she drew a short straw that she had no say in. Sam slowly moved behind me and Rocky.

My thoughts were Dana's the smallest and most nonthreatening of all of us; it could be an advantage in establishing some dialogue with the patient.

I asked Rocky to prepare Haldol, an antipsychotic medication I can give as an (intramuscular) IM injection in the upper arm. It has quick sedative effects and could help to calm her down.

Steve and Alex brought the gurney through the front door and have it ready. Now, along with Sam, they'll provide backup for Dana.

We're ready to try our plan. Dana slowly approaches Deena. We're all standing back, intently watching.

"Hi there, my name is Dana. Can you tell me your name?" Dana asked Deena with a soft and nonthreatening voice.

Deena suddenly stopped moving and tried to focus on where the voice was coming from. With her hair plastered in front of her face, she didn't have clear vision. She's also hyperactive, almost catlike with her moves, and then focuses in Dana's direction.

In the next instant, she lunged and grabbed Dana tightly around both legs just above her ankles knocking her off balance and causing her to start falling backward.

Alex was behind Dana in an instant supporting her from going back and holding her securely.

Steve and Sam are now on either side of Deena pulling at her arms trying to break her grasp of Dana.

Dana is finally able to step away and then suddenly, like a ninja, Deena is on her feet lunging at Alex, tackling him, ending up on top of him while screaming and pinning him to the floor.

This scene has eroded into a dangerous direction, and our goal is getting Deena under control without any further risk to us or her.

The officer in the kitchen has Deena by the waist and pulling her, and with Steve and Sam's help, Alex is able to get free from under her.

I have the Haldol drawn up and make my way to Deena.

"Hold her right arm still, Steve," I said.

I injected her with 10 mg of Haldol which is a large dose; we need her under control, and fast.

With Deena now on her stomach and physically restrained, she clearly isn't done struggling and continues to scream wildly.

Within a couple minutes, the Haldol is working and her activity level is waning fast.

I also decide to give her 5 mg of Ativan which is a muscle relaxer with sedative effects, and between the Haldol and Ativan, she's no longer resisting.

Steve brought the gurney over and we easily lifted her onto it and securely fastened the seat belts.

She's breathing deeply and most of all calm; we finally have the control we needed.

The crew heads to the ambulance as I'm conferring with the officers about the two kids remaining on scene.

"Their parents live a couple doors down and dispatch contacted them. They're on the way over and we'll release the kids to them," the officer said.

"Okay, well, we're going to head to RGH and hopefully have an uneventful trip," I said and headed outside.

I open the backdoor to the ambulance, and shocked to see Dana, Alex, and Sam at Deena's head. They have the bag valve mask out and providing breaths for her.

"What happened?" I asked.

"Well, we got her loaded in her, and she kind of stopped breathing, started getting blue around the lips," Sam explained.

"Okay, is air going in?" I asked.

"Oh yeah, she pinked right up with a couple breaths," Sam said.

"All right, well we better head that way," I said to Rocky.

Dana hooked up the LifePak 12 and calling out the numbers.

"Heart rate at 114, blood pressure 112/68, and SpO2 at 96%," she said.

"Those sound really good, thanks, Dana," I said.

I found a good IV site on Deena's left midarm and put a 16 gauge into it. The glucometer displays 124 for the sugar.

On reassessment, her pupils are equal and dilated which is common with hallucinogen influence; she has good chest rise, and the arm wounds are superficial.

Alex is focused on maintaining an adequate seal with the mask over Deena's mouth and nose as Sam is giving a breath every five seconds.

"You're well on your way to being our 'go to guy' for airway control," I said to Alex.

Without looking up, he nodded with a hint of vanity.

We're pulling up to RGH and Rocky parks the ambulance. Suddenly, Deena opens her eyes, and starts struggling with increasing intensity, from nothing to 100 percent just like that.

Rocky pulls the gurney and we head into the ED. Deena starts screaming at the top of her lungs, and I have no doubt they can hear her on the eighth floor.

The entire ED is looking at Deena and then me, as if I can somehow magically make this stop. Sam is trying to passively put her hand over Deena's mouth without getting bitten as we move into suite 6 and quickly have a team of nurses and Dr. Stein in the room with us.

Dr. Stein orders more Ativan; this time through the IV line which works quickly and Deena is once again somnolent.

I relay the full story, and we're happy to leave Deena in the more-than-capable hands of the RGH ED.

Out in the parking lot, we're all drained after the continual progression Deena took us through.

"See why you can't learn this stuff in the classroom?" I commented to Alex.

"I think I understand why you guys do what you do, you're good at it, and I'm still not sure how we made that work," Alex queried.

"Well, there really isn't any book, you just have to always keep the patient's best interest at the forefront, and adjust as you go," I explained.

We got back to the station and after getting everything back together and restocked, we're ready for the next one.

Alex finished his shift. He shook my hand along with the rest of the crew and left, a different person than the one who came to ride this morning.

18

OFFICER DOWN

SAM TOOK THE last two shifts off and attended a firearms competition in a neighboring county. She took second place with over one hundred contestants. The competition was fierce, and she was elated to bring her trophy in for us to see. We haven't ever seen her go below third place in these events, and she has won them on many occasions.

Our mini celebration was interrupted by the first call of the day, and tones resonating through the bay.

"Rescue 41, Medic 42, respond code three for a possible DOA, 111 Terry Place, time out 0837 hours."

Terry Place is part of a smaller neighborhood and we don't have many calls there.

We'll be on scene in less than three minutes. As we're driving up, there's a female in her fifties standing outside waving to us. The front door to the residence is open.

Rocky has the ambulance parked, and the female comes over to me as I'm exiting the vehicle.

"It's my mom, I think, I think she's dead," she said with shaky voice and lip quivering.

"Okay where is she?" I asked.

"She's in the bedroom," she said and started crying.

We grabbed the equipment and made our way into the house. The TV is on and curtains are closed. The house is immaculate and smells of lavender. The daughter isn't coming with us, and we're walking slowly down a short hallway, first peering into a room on the left and then right and then finally the last room on the right.

As we enter the room, we notice the bed has the top left corner pulled back, as if it were ready to be slept in. The pillow is without indentation. There's a small lamp on the nightstand with the light on and full glass of water next to it.

In the corner, we curiously see the patient sitting at a desk with her back to us.

There's a large mirror in front of her against the wall. She looks as if she's deep in thought, staring into it, sitting perfectly upright.

She has a pen in her right hand, posed, ready to script the next sentence. She's wearing a robe with the sleeves rolled halfway up.

For half a second, we're frozen by this presentation.

I instinctively yet meekly called out, "Hello, EMS, my name is Mark, can you hear us?"

Of course, there's no response.

I slowly approached, half expecting her to turn and acknowledge me up until the point where I checked her carotid pulse. Her skin is cool and rigor had set in. She's been dead for several hours.

She literally died and didn't move so much as an inch.

The pen in her right hand is held perfectly, barely off the paper. It's a letter she was writing to another female and had written several lines about the activities of the day, the last sentence unfinished.

This is a first for us. I wouldn't have thought this to even be possible. It's almost as if it was staged.

We now understand the shock the daughter faced as she came to check on her mother.

When we came out the house, the daughter looked at me and immediately started crying as she could tell I would confirm the news she knew, her mother was indeed dead.

"I'm so sorry," I said as I put a hand on her left shoulder.

With her hand covering her eyes, she cried openly before asking a question I have heard all too many times.

"What happened?" she asked.

"Well, I can't say for sure. It looks like she may have had a very sudden heart attack. From what we can see, it doesn't look like she had any warning or pain," I said with as much empathy as I could.

"Why's she just *sitting* there?" she asked, almost eerily.

"Well, that's kind of what I was talking about. I think whatever happened did so instantly," I said.

"I called her this morning, and she didn't answer the phone. I had a feeling something was wrong but I waited and called her again, that's when I knew," she said in between cries.

We all went into the house but she didn't go to the bedroom.

She looked around the house as if to search for some clue or answer beyond what we knew. There was nothing, everything in perfect order.

Once the deputy arrived, I explained what we had and at least gave him the warning he wouldn't find the *usual* presentation for a natural death.

I followed him back to the bedroom, and his reaction was the nearly the same as ours and he knew what to expect.

It was so surreal I checked the carotid a second time.

The daughter thanked us for coming and we cleared the scene. On the drive back to the station, Rocky and I didn't say much. I think we're both still somewhat in shock.

The rest of the morning and into the midafternoon was uneventful. Dana has a friend on another medic unit in the county and just got off the phone with her. She said they responded to a female in labor this morning and delivered a healthy baby boy at 0845.

We talked about the irony of one medic unit responding to a death while another is bringing a life in to the world. We walked away shaking our heads trying to not make too much sense of it.

Rocky was pulling the medic unit back into the bay after washing it, and Sam was finishing the rinse on the rescue when the tones had us heading to the vehicles.

"Rescue 41, Medic 42, respond code three for a motorcycle versus deer, Mile Post 4 on County Road 3, time out 1605 hours."

County Road 3 had a posted speed limit of 50 mph. We've had calls for deer strikes on this stretch of road. In a vehicle, it can be dangerous; on a motorcycle, it can be deadly.

We're met by traffic backed up for almost a quarter mile prior to the crash. It has lanes blocked in both directions as evidenced by no traffic coming at us.

Our response took six minutes.

A deputy is waving to us and standing next to the patient who's lying face down. There's a massive pool of blood surrounding his head.

The motorcycle is fifty feet further down the road. The front wheel is bent indicating this may have been a head on collision with the animal.

A large deer is lying on the opposite side of the road, and mercifully DOA with its neck grotesquely twisted and blood streaming from its nose.

Sam and Dana are going to the patient's head. We can hear breathing with interposed gurgling and an occasional moan.

He's wearing a small skullcap-type helmet which mostly protects only the back of the head.

With the patient in the prone position, face down, we can't effectively secure his airway or properly assess him.

A quick check of his back doesn't reveal any injuries.

As Dana holds the patient's head in line, she calls out the roll as Rocky has the spine board next to him.

"One, two, three, roll," she directed and he's secure to the spine board.

As soon as we have him supine, face up, he begins to have immediate airway issues, choking, gagging.

This is secondary to the massive injuries to his face that make him nearly unrecognizable as a person.

We then notice the heavy bruising to the front of his neck. It's deformed and when it's felt; there are rice krispies throughout the neck up toward the ear.

He has a fractured trachea. This is a major finding and will require immediate attention.

He's covered in blood and fur. It's difficult to know if the blood is his or the deer's. We know who the fur belongs to.

His eyes are swollen shut with periorbital ecchymosis surrounding them; he has a full-thickness laceration above the left brow with shiny white skull exposed. His nose resembles the letter "S" and steady bleeding from both nares. His top lip is torn near the left corner exposing the gumline and several teeth are missing or broken.

I've never seen a fractured trachea. This is a rare injury and can be difficult to manage.

I listen to breath sounds and hear air equally on both sides. Steve is cutting clothing which includes protective leather coat and pants.

Sam and Dana are working feverishly trying to keep this airway open and clear of the blood draining into the back of his throat.

Dana has a large trauma dressing over the left side of the forehead and secured. When she's gently applying direct pressure to the lacerated lip, we notice the lower jaw is in several pieces.

Sam is using the suction and oxygen mask at the same time, and the patient is still developing circumoral cyanosis, blueness around the mouth.

Rocky tossed me two rubber tourniquets, and I put one on each upper arm in hope of having a vein pop up by the time we get into the ambulance.

After seven minutes on scene, we're heading to RGH.

Dana has the LifePak 12 hooked up and calling out the first numbers.

"Heart rate 128, blood pressure 80/68, and SpO2 is 86%," she said.

I found a large vein in the left midarm and put a 14 gauge in. I'm ready to begin the RSI procedure and secure this airway. I changed places with Sam and prepared for the intubation.

"Sam, put the cricothyrotomy kit on the counter," I said as Sam looked at Dana and both had serious looks about them.

This would be the first time I've called for it to be close.

With the fractured trachea, trauma to the mouth and blood obscuring the field of view, this will be a difficult intubation. We didn't have any other choice. We're having trouble keeping his oxygen level high enough, and he's at risk for vomiting and aspiration.

These are the tough decisions a paramedic will make, and live with.

I nodded to Dana and the RSI drugs went in one after the other. The patient stopped breathing, no turning back now. I introduced the blade down his throat and almost immediately needed suction.

Sam is an outline of me trying to get the same view I have and staying a step in front of me clearing the way. I finally get to the back of the throat and the blood flow is overwhelming us. I've lost all landmarks; all I can see is blood, swollen tissue, and two of the missing teeth.

"Heart rate dropping, SpO2 at 70%," Dana called out with heightened concern.

This is a worst-case scenario. He's becoming critically hypoxic (oxygen depleted) and in danger of going into cardiac arrest.

I have no choice but to abandon the attempt and get him oxygenated.

Dana rolled the long spine board toward her and braced it against her hips while staring intently at the LifePak 12. This will help with secretions that are going down the throat.

Sam is aligning the jaw with both hands while holding the bag valve between her knees as I am sealing the mask over his mouth and nose.

Between the dressings, loose tissues and bleeding, we're at the bottom of our "bag of tricks."

Her legs go together squeezing the bag valve. Blood sprays wildly on the first attempt.

"Heart rate 40 and SpO2 60%," Dana called out, this time with no doubt what's coming next.

The intensity of the moment is palpable. This guy is seconds away from coding!

After a reposition of the jaw by Sam and mask by me, her legs go together a second time squeezing the bag and chest rises, another squeeze, chest rise, another and then another.

"Heart rate coming up, 90, and SpO2 at 84%," Dana called out.

After several more leg squeezes of bag, I'm ready to try for the second attempt at the intubation. I'm also running out of time as the RSI drugs will start to wear off, and his gag reflex will return making the intubation all but impossible.

I have one last shot before having to use the cricothyrotomy kit.

For this next attempt, I am having Sam employ the fishhook maneuver, which created the larger mouth opening along with strategically using the suction.

This philosophy is a trick of the trade; if it didn't work the first time, don't try it a second time, and come up with a new plan.

As I get to the tracheal opening, I reach to the front of his neck and gently move the structure to the right, now I have a perfect view.

"Sam, put your left hand right where mine is and hold it," I said.

With her right hand holding the mouth open, her left hand snaked between my arms stabilizing the throat, right leg bent beneath her on the jump seat and crouching with her left leg, she looks like a contortionist performing her climatic finish.

I breathe a sigh of relief as I watch the end of the endotracheal tube go through the red-stained vocal cords and into the trachea.

Sam whispered aloud, "Yes, I felt it pass by my fingers."

"Roger that," I replied back as we lightly bumped heads in triumph.

Sam sat in a more relaxed position in the jump seat as she attached the bag valve to the end of the tube, and after a couple of squeezes, we see good chest rise, his color is back to pink, we have an airway.

"Heart rate at 126, blood pressure 84/60, and SpO2 at 92%," Dana called out with obvious elation.

I offered her a look of relief as I picked up the cricothyrotomy kit and put it back on the shelf.

He must have taken the deer face first for this degree of injury. This guy is far from being out of danger; we've only bought him time.

We're two minutes from RGH and the trauma team is standing by. We have plenty of help as we arrive and directed to suite 12.

Dr. Robertson, trauma surgeon, is leading the team and pace is blistering. There are labs being drawn and x-rays and notes being made. The decision is made to go to the OR for repair of the trachea and facial injuries.

We learned our patient's name is Phillip. He's twenty-four years old and a student at the community college. After several hours in the OR, he's admitted to the trauma ICU.

One of his x-rays showed three teeth in the stomach.

The RSI procedure is a lifesaving option for the critically ill or injured patient. It's an extremely invasive procedure and isn't without significant risk involved; 99.9 percent of the cases are uneventful and quickly successful.

When you personally experience the 0.1 percent with complications, the world seems to stop; it's up there at one of the most stresses any EMS provider can want to face.

Like Dr. Stein says, "When you work with good folks, you get good results."

My crew is the epitome of that passage.

Two weeks had passed since we transported Phillip to the hospital. We followed his progress and made it to the ICU to briefly talk with him.

He can only speak in a soft whisper and it's chilling to hear his account.

He recalls the deer jumping into the road and describes himself and the deer as being face to face and *eye to eye*. Then, smelling its breath is the last thing he remembers until waking in the ICU forty-eight hours later.

His face is a road map of sutures and rainbow of colors: red, purple, yellow, and blue. He faces months of reconstructive surgeries, literally. He does however have a story that will be hard to beat at family gatherings.

It's Wednesday afternoon and the day has been busy with three minor medical calls and two minor traffic crashes. We haven't seen much of the station. Our home away from home has been the ED EMS break room. It's a day of graham crackers, strawberry, and vanilla yogurt and peel back top juice drinks—the EMS version of gourmet fine dining.

Getting back to the station for dinner will be a treat. We're in the kitchen preparing for chicken burgers, fries, and raisin oatmeal cookies Rachel sent to work with Rocky for the crew. This will be our weekly off-the-diet meal.

The tones would ensure this meal would become a late-night snack.

"Rescue 41, Medic 42, Medic 32, respond code three for an officer involved shooting, multiple patients, officer down, 9460 Oakmont Street, time out 1820 hours."

We made it to the rigs and out the door quickly. The dispatch sounded ominous. This was outside of our primary response area and in District 3's stomping grounds.

We'll be second ambulance in which means we'd get the most critical patient. "First in, last out" was the saying.

The first unit on scene would conduct the triage. They would prioritize the patients according to severity. The second ambulance in would take the most critical and, "load and go," which will be us.

There's a lot of police activity on the scanner. It sounds like they have control and requesting EMS respond directly into the scene.

Medic 32 checked out and we waited for their size up. It's Holly Ryan and came in less than a minute.

"Medic 42 and Rescue 41 from Medic 32...be advised we have two patients, your patient will be the suspect, he has multiple gunshot wounds to the chest, come in off 94th," she said.

Steve and I both copied the update.

"I'm going to get things set up in the back," I told Rocky.

"Roger that, hang on," he said.

I crawled through the walkway into the patient compartment and got two IVs set up, plugged the cables into the LifePak 12, set out airway equipment, and grabbed two rubber tourniquets. As usual, I will put one on each of the patient's arms as we make contact.

We arrived in the middle of at least a dozen patrol cars. The scene is still active and lots of big guns being carried.

We see the Medic 32 crew directly in front of us in the next block. There's a car broadsided around a utility pole where it hit driver's door first. The passenger door is open.

Off to the side of the wrecked car is a patrol car with the driver's door open. The backside window is shattered and several bullet holes in the side of the patrol car.

We would learn the driver of the crashed car drew the attention of the patrol officer as he went through a red light.

The patrol officer followed the car for a short distance and initiated a traffic stop. A brief high-speed chase ended as the suspect lost control and broadsided the pole.

He exited the passenger side, pistol in hand, firing wildly on the patrol car and officer. The officer returned fire and suspect was shot twice in the chest and once in the leg.

The officer was hit once in the left leg. He's standing between two officers in front of another patrol car and being treated by Tony, the EMT from Medic 32.

Our patient is face down, handcuffed behind his back. He's squirming, agitated, and looking around, almost hyperactive.

Holly Ryan is the paramedic from Medic 32. We haven't seen her since we got hit on the freeway last month.

As I walk toward her, she smiles, "Hey, Mark, this is your patient and as you can see he isn't real happy right now. He has two in the right chest, one high, one low, and one in the right thigh, he has a radial pulse at a buck twenty, absent breath sounds on the upper right and that's as far as we got. This officer is going with you," she said.

"Okay, thanks, Holly, we'll see you at the hospital," I said.

She smiled, pointed at Sam, and turned away.

Steve started cutting the patient's clothes off. He has to avoid cutting through bullet entry holes as the clothing will be used as reconstructive evidence.

Rocky has the long spine board ready. I put a rubber tourniquet on both upper arms. Now we need to get the patient secured to the spine board, on his back. This will be a challenge as the officers will be hesitant to remove his handcuffs. I understand this is a very bad guy, but right now I have only one focus and that's get him to the hospital alive.

Several officers assist us and he is quickly secured and handcuffed to the spine board.

There are two good-sized holes in his chest. He was hit three times with a 9mm.

The first one is just below the right clavicle, collarbone. It's about the size of a quarter and bleeding is minimal. The second hole is a couple inches below the right nipple and also about the size of a quarter. It's bleeding is a steady flow and has a deep purple hue to it.

There are no exit wounds.

Dana has two occlusive dressings over the wounds and taped in place. A quick listen to the chest with the stethoscope reveals the decreased breath sounds in the right upper fields as Holly mentioned.

The hole in the right upper thigh is perfect center. I believe it hit the femur. There's no exit. Steve wrapped it with a large trauma dressing and taped it tightly.

We're on scene for four minutes from the time we made patient contact. Sam's at the patient's head and has an oxygen mask over his mouth and nose.

He continues to squirm and resist our efforts. In fact, he can be classified as a combative patient which is any patient resisting treatment, regardless of their injury or illness.

We have his head taped to the spine board and cervical collar in place. Sam is challenged with keeping him from lifting his head up. He's becoming more enraged by the second.

Dana has the LifePak 12 hooked up and has the first readings.

"Heart rate 140, blood pressure 80/54, and he won't leave the SpO2 clip on his finger," she called out.

I have two good IV sites in the left arm. I put a 14 gauge in the upper site. I'm going to put him asleep with the RSI procedure and take control of his airway.

This will also prevent him from the potential to do more harm to himself with his injuries. I have the drugs drawn and going to switch places with Sam.

The patient makes eye contact with me and fights violently against his restraints; he manages to slide his oxygen mask off.

With a loud and exaggerated deep clearing of his throat, he spits a thick wad of phlegm hitting the left side of my head with a resounding thud.

Sam pulls his head back down and puts the oxygen mask back over his face.

The officer makes a move toward the patient as I put my hand up and said, "It's all right, we got him," and closed my eyes for a second trying not to think about what just happened.

Dana reaches up with a trauma dressing and cleans the side of my head.

I have no choice but to stay focused on what needs to be done. I give Dana the go ahead to start the RSI drugs, and within seconds the patient is unconscious and stopped breathing.

"Did he just die?" the officer asked.

"Well, no, we just put him asleep and now we're going to intubate him and breathe for him," I said.

After slowly sliding the laryngoscope blade down his throat, I have a good view of the vocal cords. The tube is advanced past the cords, and now Sam is ventilating him.

I need to get him reassessed.

His pupils are dilated, large. We see this sometimes secondary to methamphetamine influence.

The right chest still has decreased breath sounds but no signs of building tension. The dressing over the lower chest wound is soaked with blood and I place a second one over the top of it. The right leg dressing is holding. I put a second IV in the left arm in the lower site.

"Heart rate 145, blood pressure 74/46, and SpO2 84%," Dana called out.

Are we going to lose this guy? I wondered.

After updating RGH with the latest information, we have a reservation with suite 12.

The trauma team sprung into high gear, and after an x-ray, the patient is off the OR. Both bullets are still in his chest.

After nearly two hours and multiple units of blood, he's admitted to the trauma ICU in critical condition under heavy police guard. The bullet in the right upper chest did extensive damage along with having the right upper lobe of the lung removed.

The lower wound did extensive damage to the liver and bowel.

The thigh wound shattered the femur and will be repaired after he's stabilized.

The suspect is nineteen years old and has an extensive arrest record for drug-related crimes. He tested positive for near-critical levels of methamphetamine and cocaine, plus an alcohol level of .24.

If the suspect survives and makes it to court, we'll all be subpoenaed to testify about our roles in the case. We will see him again.

The officer he shot was treated and released after treatment for a through-and-through (gunshot wound) GSW to the left thigh.

We've said it and thought it many times; we wouldn't trade what we do with anyone, ever. We're exactly where we're all supposed to be.

...and Dana ate more than her share of raisin oatmeal cookies later.

EPILOGUE

EMS HAS BEEN around in some form or another since the beginning of mankind. It may not have been known as EMS in those early days of man's existence, but the desire to help another fellow human being is ingrained in all of us. We see examples of this play out almost every day where a random person comes to the aid of someone in trouble. Then there are those individuals who take it to the next level and dedicate their lives to bringing comfort to suffering and order out of chaos.

Being part of this delivery system has been a privilege and experience I couldn't have imagined. When I first got into EMS, I was told to expect an average of a five-year career. I certainly didn't look at it that way and over thirty years later I look forward to being part of the EMS world every day and proud of it.

The bonds formed between the crews become very strong. The emotions, the sights, the sounds, the personal experiences, the humorous moments, the tragedies, the saves, and the inevitable part of death and dying, all of it can sculpt us to become part of the EMS brotherhood we all share.

We're not invulnerable. Being part of EMS can toll great sacrifice on personal relationships and families. The missed holidays, birthdays, and special events because mom or dad was on shift.

We believe we *can* make a difference on each and every call we respond to. We're bringing the best of the best. We also employ the most aggressive patient care guidelines along with the latest and most sophisticated equipment. Our edge is our experience and strong desire to change the odds in our favor, and we do this quite regularly.

The stories in *Signs of Life II* are based on real events over the last thirty years. Steve, Sam, Dana, Rocky, Joe, and Brandon, along with all the others, are based on partners and crews I've had the honor of working with. I would need an entire separate book to recognize the hundreds of professionals I've been privileged to be associated with. The patient names and some scenarios have been altered to protect the confidentiality of not only the patient but also families of the patients.

The average family will never experience the tragedies we can be involved in on any given day. But when a family is faced with an event that will change their lives forever, we become part of that and have an opportunity to give them a starting point for healing that can take years or even a lifetime.

One morning, we came on duty and were dispatched to a DOA. After we arrived, it was quickly determined there wasn't anything we could do. The male had died during the night and had been dead for several hours. The wife was devastated, inconsolable, and paralyzed with fear. We ended up spending hours at the home with her until we eventually were able to contact her son and he came to the house. We didn't realize it at the time, but our efforts were what got her through those first few hours and then days of accepting she was alone.

Several years later, my partner and I were eating at a restaurant. We were aware an elderly lady kept smiling at us. When we left she followed us out into the parking lot. It was the lady we had spent the time with after her husband died. She thanked us for that morning and how it helped her beyond words. She created a bereavement group that's still active today, and we gave her the inspiration for forming this chapter.

We don't get into EMS for the recognition and certainly not for the fortune. I wouldn't trade the experiences for anything. I'm proud to share these stories and do so with humbled and respectful intention.

Now, hug your significant other and tell them it's for "no reason," hug your child and smile at them every day, call your friend, talk to your neighbor, tell them how much you appreciate their friendship and most of all, look in the mirror and tell *that* person how special *they* are.

Also, remember, you *do* make a difference in someone's life, *every* day.

Thanks for riding with us and being part of these experiences; we enjoyed having you.

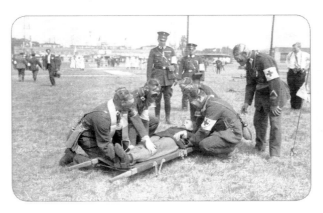

Early EMS and proof it's been around in some form or another in every century and culture. (Am I the only one who has about ten questions I'd like to ask about this scene?)
From April 1931

GLOSSARY

A

ABCs. This is airway, breathing and circulation. We conduct a primary and secondary survey for all patients. The ABCs is the *primary*. This rapidly ensures the patient has a patent airway, effective breathing, and adequate pulse. We'll evaluate these more in-depth along with everything else in the *secondary* survey. In the public setting, they're now advocating hands only CPR, not worrying about spending time checking the ABCs.

ACLS. This is advanced cardiac life support. It's a two-year certification that guides the clinician in treatment for cardiac emergencies, cardiac arrest, acute myocardial infarction, or AMI (heart attack) and strokes at the advanced level. The precursor to initiating ACLS is BCLS, basic cardiac life support, or CPR. The saying is, "Good BCLS compliments good ACLS," and patients have better outcomes. It is a sixteen-hour class broken in to two eight-hour days with lecture and practical scenarios.

agonal respiration. This is higher brain activity that kicks in after a person goes into cardiac arrest. Agonal means "dying." The body continues to simulate breathing when in reality there's no actual oxygen exchange. It can be mistaken for breathing and the lay rescuer will be hesitant to begin CPR. The clue is unresponsiveness and color of the patient, blue and ashen, and they'll look dead. If you error on the side of helping them and they wake up, this is a good thing because it means they're alive.

agonal rhythm. This is a presentation on the cardiac monitor that's an ominous development. There is no pulse associated with this showing. The heart produces a natural electrical impulse that's captured on the EKG screen. When the body runs out of blood, this electrical activity continues to show up. The EKG rhythm doesn't look like the normal EKG rhythm with the regularly spaced up and down tracings. It's bizarre, wide, and looks bad. In general, this presentation has poor resuscitation success rates.

anaphylactic shock. This is an exaggerated response to an allergic reaction. Common allergies include bee stings, peanuts, shellfish, and some medications. During anaphylactic shock, the blood pressure drops, the smaller airways in the lungs constrict and swelling can occur in the throat with complete airway loss. Any person suspected of having an allergic reaction needs immediate evaluation by EMS. People who've had severe reactions might carry an EpiPen or auto-injector. You can assist a person having an emergency with their auto-injector but *never* use it on them without their permission or if they're unconscious. And certainly *never* use it on someone else.

angina pectoris. This is a form of heart disease. It's specifically a narrowing at some point in the coronary arteries. These are the arteries that supply the heart muscle itself with blood and life-sustaining oxygen. When the flow is restricted, the heart responds with some variation of pain; squeezing, sharp, dull, heavy, crushing, or a burning sensation that can be mistaken for heartburn. Patients with diagnosed angina might carry nitroglycerin tablets or spray. When they have angina-type pain, they use the medication and it specifically dilates or makes the coronary artery bigger and allows more blood to reach the oxygen-deprived cardiac tissue. If someone is having this pain, you can assist them with the nitro administration, but *never* give it to them without their request or if they're unconscious or use it on someone else.

anoxia. This is medical terminology that means without oxygen. *An*=without, *oxia*=oxygen.

appears. This is a word that should never be used in your EMS chart. It means "you don't know." Write what you see.

aspiration. This is any foreign substance that's inhaled into the lungs. It can be liquid or solid. This includes vomiting, drowning, food, etc. This is one of the reasons we'll RSI a patient that's unconscious. Once they're intubated, their airway and lungs are protected from this potentiality. See RSI

asystole. This is flatline on the EKG screen, no electrical activity in the heart. We *do not* shock this rhythm despite them shocking it on TV and miraculously getting the heart started again. We've treated cardiac arrests where families got upset because we didn't shock their loved one and complained because, "They do it on TV and it saves them."

Ativan. This is a muscle relaxant and antianxiety medication; we use it in several different instances. It can be used for sedation, and sometimes during a painful procedure such as applying a traction splint on a femur fracture on a conscious person. It can be given IV or IM.

B

bag valve mask. Used for delivering breaths to a person not breathing or needing assisted breathing. It consists of a self-inflating football-shaped rubber bag with a mask which fits over the mouth and nose. It can be used by one or two persons. The optimal use is by two people; one will squeeze the bag while the other will hold the mask over the mouth and nose making an adequate seal. Once a patient is intubated, the mask part is no longer needed. The bag valve will attach to the endotracheal tube and breaths are delivered straight into the lungs.

Benadryl. A medication we use during an allergic reaction in combination with epinephrine. Benadryl relieves the itching and hives. Hives are red blots all over the chest, back, and arms. The medical word for hives is *urticaria* and itching is *pruritus*. Benadryl is an (over-the-counter) OTC medication also known as diphenhydramine.

big needle. This is one of the extreme event items and used to relieve a tension pneumothorax. It's a 12 gauge, three-inch long needle. It's called the *big needle* because it is a big needle.

blown pupil. This is unequal pupils; one is of normal size while the other is dilated or large. The patient is generally *not* conscious with this presentation. It's associated with serious rising intracranial pressure. There's usually some significant (mechanism of injury) MOI involved like a recent head injury or some major insult to the brain. Blown pupil is the slang term.

breath sounds. This is a shortened phrase that indicates assessment of the chest with a stethoscope. We're looking for equality, wheezing such as with asthma, fluid sounds which indicates some type of heart failure or maybe drowning. With a trauma patient, this assessment should happen fairly quickly.

A way to chart this is, "BS are clear and equal bilaterally." The "BS" stands for breath sounds and "bilaterally" referring to both sides.

BVM. This is the abbreviation for bag valve mask.

C

cardiac alert. This is a term we'll advise the receiving hospital of. It's a patient that fits criteria for immediate cardiac evaluation on arrival to the emergency department and could be a candidate for the catheterization lab or clot busting medication to resolve the blocked coronary arteries or even bypass surgery. The prehospital philosophy is, "Time is muscle." We base this alert on the specific complaint, physical findings like the 12-lead EKG along with past medical history and risk factors like smoking, high blood pressure, diabetes, obesity, etc.

CCU. This is the coronary care unit. When you have a cardiac emergency you'll end up here after being stabilized in the ED or the cath lab or maybe even the OR. After you're stabilized from here, they'll transfer you to a medical floor before being discharged home.

circumoral cyanosis. This is medical terminology that means blueness around the lips from lack of oxygen. We see it in asthmatics, emphysema, and in trauma with pneumothorax and any condition that makes the person hypoxic, low on oxygen. *Circum*=around, *oral*=mouth, *cyan*=blue, *osis*= condition.

clavicle. This is the collarbone. This bone is a reference point for inserting the big needle during a tension pneumothorax. It's inserted between the second and third ribs, midline with the clavicle.

clinically dead. You're clinically dead the second your pulse stops. Without treatment and restoration of a heartbeat, you will become biologically dead after several minutes. Clinical death requires immediate CPR. The local newspaper did an article about us one day and got this terminology mixed up. The headline for the article read: Paramedics Revive Biologically Dead Man.

coded. This term is used to indicate a patient has gone into cardiac arrest. Someone monitoring a patient and their EKG would shout out, "He just coded," and this will bring the resuscitation team. At this point, the patient is clinically dead, no pulse. There's a trauma code, which the patient has coded from trauma. Trauma code resuscitations have very poor outcomes.

code three. This is driving with overhead lights and siren activated. It's an extremely dangerous mode of travel as you never know what can be around the next corner or what the driver in front of you will do. The odds of being involved in a vehicle crash are greatly increased when operating in this mode. It requires complete attention from not only the driver but also from your partner as well. Four eyes are better than two. It's not a free pass to drive like a maniac or out of control or satisfy pent-up road rage hostilities. It's essentially a way of politely asking drivers to yield the right of way. EMS personnel have been put in jail after crashes while operating the ambulance in this mode and found at fault. The public can reduce this risk by paying attention and yielding the right of way when approached by an ambulance with lights and siren.

combative patient. This is a term we can use to describe the activity level of a patient that is less than cooperative toward treatment. It can be drug or alcohol related. It can have legitimate medical causes as well, insulin shock, postictal after a seizure, disoriented. It can be a very difficult patient to deal with as they may be going full throttle at fighting you and you have to use restraint.

combo-pads. Rectangular pads with strong adhesive backing that stick firmly to the patient's chest used to monitor the EKG rhythm and deliver a shock during cardiac arrest. There are small wires from each pad and attachment that plugs into the LifePak 12. One pad is placed on the upper chest above the right nipple and the other on the lower chest below the left nipple. On patients who have a thick *carpet* or *rug* of chest hair, we use a disposable razor to *trim* the area to ensure the pad makes good contact with the skin and reduce the risk of an out-of-control *chest hair fire.*

cricothyrotomy kit. This is a kit used to make a surgical opening at the cricothyroid membrane in the front of the neck. It creates a temporary airway during a traumatic or catastrophic medical emergency where an airway cannot be obtained by, head-tilt chin lift, jaw thrust, BVM, or intubation. It's also one of the five extreme event items.

crow's foot laceration. This is a laceration that resembles a crow's foot. It's usually above the eye and full thickness meaning it's fairly deep. If you ever see one, you'll look at it and think, "That looks like a crow's foot!" After it is sutured the patient does fine.

CT scan. This is computed tomography. It's a detailed sectional view of the body part or area that's being evaluated. It's useful for assessing head injuries and not used in the prehospital arena, yet.

cyanosis. This is blueness to the skin and secondary to lack of oxygen carried in the red blood cells. It's a frightening presentation. The initial treatment is to provide supplemental oxygen and then correct the underlying cause.

D

defibrillate. This is delivering a shock to ventricular fibrillation which is cardiac arrest, no pulse, along with CPR. The goal is to stop the fibrillating activity or knock it out, and then allow the heart to restart on its own. The movies have portrayed this as jump-starting the heart which is the opposite of what really happens. The operator needs to ensure no one is touching the patient during the delivery of the shock or they could receive part of the energy, thus the chant, "Clear."

D50. This is a medication we give someone with a low blood sugar that's either unconscious or too obtunded to take in food or sugar orally, or by mouth. It's a concentrated bolus of sugar water that's administered through the IV line. It rapidly raises the blood sugar levels and wakes them immediately from insulin shock. It's important they eat something afterward as the bolus will not stay in the system for very long.

dextrose 50%. This is D50.

DOA. Dead on Arrival—not something you want written in your medical record.

E

ecchymosis. This is medical terminology for bluish discoloration, like a bruise. Periorbital ecchymosis means a black eye. Ecchymosis is the discoloration part.

EKG. This is the electrocardiogram. It might be called the ECG or EKG, either term is used. It's the viewing of electrical activity of the heart displayed on the screen. It's not a reflection of what's actually going on in the body. You still need to assess for actual pulses and blood pressure and level of consciousness.

Elavil. This is an antidepressant medication. Overdose can cause major cardiac abnormalities, dangerously low blood pressure, and if untreated, death. There is no antidote. We call this group of medication TCAs—tricyclic antidepressants.

emphysema. This is a progressive airway disease that involves the small air sacs where oxygen exchange occurs in the lungs. These little sacs are called alveoli and the disease causes destructive changes to the walls of these structures. The patient may eventually need to be on oxygen full time. It has been linked to smoking.

EMS. This is the emergency medical services abbreviation. It covers all aspects of the prehospital care arena. It would take pages and pages to adequately do justice to describing this organization and its progressive mission.

endotracheal tube. This is a long plastic tube inserted orally (into the mouth) and into the trachea during the intubation process. The portion sticking out of the mouth will be attached to the bag valve in order for breaths to be given. This is part of the ultimate protection of an airway a patient cannot protect themselves. These are people that are unconscious, severe trauma, facial burns, etc.

epidural bleed. This is bleeding in a layer of the brain. It is a collection of blood just under the skull. *Epi*=on top of, *dura*=the outer layer of the brain. This person may have a decrease in their mentation or be unconscious. This also qualifies as a (traumatic brain injury) TBI. Epidural bleeds are generally suspected in patient's that receive a blow to the side of the head.

epiglottis. This is the flap in the back of the throat that sits above the tracheal opening. Not the little punching bag that's visible with the mouth open, which is the uvula. The epiglottis is further down and a landmark during the intubation process. Once we see this, we know the tracheal opening is just beneath it.

epinephrine. This is a medication used during cardiac arrest to stimulate activity and for anaphylactic shock. In cardiac arrest, it's given intravenously or IV. For anaphylactic shock, it's given as an IM injection. People with severe allergies and at risk for anaphylactic shock will carry an EpiPen and inject this into their lateral thigh and through clothing during an emergency. A bystander can assist this person but should *never* administer it without their consent.

ETA. This is the estimated time of arrival.

etomidate. This is a medication we use during the RSI procedure. It induces anesthesia or deep sleep and is a powerful amnesiac mercifully giving the person going through the procedure the benefit of having no memory of it.

extreme event items. These are the five items used during extreme events and warrant everyone on the crew knowing their location and complete understanding on using them. They consist of: 1-The big needle, 12 gauge-three-inch catheter used for tension pneumothorax, 2-The OB kit, 3-The burn sheets, 4-The cricothyrotomy kit, and 5-The 10 × 30-inch trauma dressings.

F

fishhook method. This is a trick to gain an advantage during the intubation process on someone with a small mouth opening. An assistant will use one finger, generally the right index finger and pull the patient's right cheek out to the side and thereby increasing the size of the opening to the mouth, allowing more room to insert the endotracheal tube. The assistant has to work in conjunction with the person performing the intubation and not just pull blindly.

G

glucometer. Small handheld device used for measuring blood glucose levels in the blood. Normal readings are 70–110 mg/dL. We have two ways to elicit the blood sample needed for the measurement. One is using blood from the IV needle after the IV is established. The other is to use a small lancet and prick a finger drawing a small amount of blood. If this method is used we'll use the lateral (side) portion of the finger as opposed to the pad (front). The lateral side of the finger is less painful.

go big or go home. This is a saying in EMS, it refers to establishing the biggest IV possible in your trauma patient. If you're the patient, and you hear this, you know you're getting a large IV.

grand mal seizure. This is violent uncoordinated muscle contractions secondary to brain activity. There are many reasons for the seizure including epilepsy, low blood sugar, low oxygen levels, high fever, head injuries, tumors, and sometimes no cause found. It's important to protect the person having the seizure from harm; placing something soft under their head to prevent them from banging their head against a hard surface can prevent a secondary head injury. *Do not* physically restrain them as this can cause injury. *Do not* put anything in their mouth during the seizure. Once the seizure has stopped, check their breathing and ensure 9-1-1 has been called.

GSW. Gunshot wound.

H

Haldol. This is an antipsychotic medication we use for acute psychotic episodes, it has sedative effects and can be given IV or IM.

hematoma. This is a collection of blood under the skin making a bluish discoloration. In EMS slang, it is also called a "hema-tomatoe."

heroin. This is an illegal narcotic and highly addictive. It's an opiate derivative. Overdoses suppress the receptor sites in the body that measure rising carbon dioxide levels and you just fail to breathe. If the person isn't discovered within a couple minutes, cardiac arrest ensues and they die. The drug can be injected, snorted, and smoked. We see increases in overdoses when a new shipment of the drug comes to town in stronger concentrations than users are accustomed to.

humerus. This is the upper arm bone and one of two long bones in the human skeleton. The other long bone is the femur. Both of these bones require great force to fracture.

hypoxia. This is medical terminology meaning low oxygen state. The patient may have secondary cyanosis, blueness along with it. *Hypo*=low, *oxia*=oxygen.

I

ICU. This is the intensive care unit. After you are stabilized, in either the ED or after the operating room, you're sent to the ICU where you get more intensive care and monitoring. After you're stabilized in the ICU, you're transferred to a medical floor before being discharged home.

IM/intramuscular. This is a shot like you would get at the doctor's office or clinic. IM stands for intramuscular. It's generally given in the upper arm. It's not a quick way to get a drug into the system, IV is the quickest. When we give something in the IM route, we can only hope it gets into the system quickly.

incontinence. This is an involuntary release of the urinary bladder. We may see this when someone has been unconscious or after a grand mal seizure. Sometimes, we'll arrive at a trauma scene and the patient is awake. We notice they have a wet spot, and this tells us they may have lost consciousness prior to our arrival even though they're not aware of it.

insulin. This is a medication taken by diabetics with a nonfunctioning pancreas and inability to produce insulin. Insulin is needed to control blood sugar levels. Taken regularly with a proper diet, blood sugar levels stay in check. If a diabetic uses insulin and fails to eat, the sugar level will drop, and they can become unconscious and this is known as insulin shock.

insulin shock. This is too much insulin. The patient will have an altered mentation and can go downhill very quickly. The lay public will sometimes call this a diabetic coma, which is actually the opposite, extremely high blood sugar. For the insulin shock, we need to get an IV started on them and administer D50 which wakes them rapidly. They then eat a carbohydrate meal to sustain the sugar levels.

intubation. This is a procedure that secures the airway with an endotracheal tube. Any patient that cannot actively control their own airway is at risk for aspiration and hypoxia. It's considered the gold standard for protecting the airway.

IV. This means intravenously, in to the vein. We place plastic IV catheters into the veins to administer fluids and/or medications. The largest IV catheter we can place in a vein is a 14 gauge. A small IV would be a 20 gauge. The smaller the number, the larger the catheter is. In trauma, we use the larger catheters. "Go big or go home."

J

jaw thrust. Method used to open an airway with suspected cervical spine injury. The patient who needs this will make snoring sounds indicating the tongue is creating a partial obstruction of the airway. The jaw thrust brings the tongue forward and relieves this condition. It's easiest to perform this maneuver from the top of the patient's head, using both hands along the jaw line and with the index fingers used to gently displace the jaw in a forward motion. If someone is snoring and keeping the household awake, this maneuver will work; unfortunately you won't get any sleep, but you won't have to listen to that noise any longer.

joules. This is one of two terms used to describe the energy delivered during ventricular fibrillation. One is joules and the other is watt seconds. They're both measurement of energies. We might start at 200 joules and progress to a maximum of 360 joules. We'll generally just call out a number when on scene and leave the joules or watt seconds part off.

K

KISS theory. Keep It Simple, Stupid. This acronym is used in many circles, but I believe it may have originated in EMS; it certainly fits us, "Keep it simple, stupid, it's not that hard."

L

laryngoscope blade. These are long stainless steel blades with a light on the end that's attached to the laryngoscope handle. It's used during the intubation process. There are two basic designs—a straight blade and curved blade. Other names for the blades are Miller (straight blade) and Macintosh (curved). Most paramedics have their own preference on which blade they will start with. My preference is the Mac 4. You should be proficient with using both blades.

laryngoscope handle. The laryngoscope blade is attached to the laryngoscope handle. The handle is stainless steel and contains two "C" cell batteries.

level one trauma center. This is a hospital capable of delivering the highest level of care, 24-7 and 365 days a year.

LifePak 12. This is our cardiac or heart monitor. It's capable of monitoring the electrical rhythm of the heart and displays this on a large screen. It can print a copy of what we see which is included in our documentation of the incident. It's also used to shock, or defibrillate at patient in cardiac arrest with ventricular fibrillation, it can pace a slow heart and speed it up, and it can take automatic blood pressures and monitor the SpO2 or oxygen levels in the blood.

LPN. This is a licensed practical nurse.

M

MAST. This is the medical antishock trousers. They started out as military antishock trousers as it was developed by the military to prevent pilots from blacking out during high-speed maneuvers in fighter jets. It was then used for traumatically injured soldiers with primary blood loss, the theory being it would squeeze blood from the legs and pelvis to the core area where it would be more beneficial until surgical intervention. We primarily use them now for stabilizing and splinting closed lower extremity (femur) and pelvic fractures. It's a tough nylon suit of pants and pelvic section that's placed on a patient like a pair of pants, and then external hoses introduce air into bladders sewn into the fabric which becomes tight around the legs and pelvis. You can inflate each section individually if needed.

methamphetamine. An illegal street drug classified as a stimulant. It's manufactured illegally in meth labs set up in homes, cars, and under extremely dangerous conditions and highly addictive. It can have adverse effects to the heart, brain, and cause death. The user will have dilated or large pupils, be sweaty, and tweaks, unable to remain still, smacking the lips, and can stay awake for days.

MDT. These are mobile data terminals. They're mounted to the dash in the ambulance and a link to the dispatch center. They're about the size of a laptop. We can receive updated information about the call we're responding to.

medic unit. This is another term for the ambulance. You may hear people also refer to it as the bus. I believe this is a derogatory term although it's popular with many EMS responders.

MHP. This is a mental health professional. They can assess and recommend treatment for patients having acute psychological problems.

MICP. This is an acronym for mobile intensive care paramedic; as in Mark Mosier, Joey Capthorn, or Eric Wright.

MICU. This is an acronym for mobile intensive care unit, our office.

morphine. This is a potent narcotic pain reliever. It's an opiate derivative. We administer it intravenously or IV. It has the potential to interfere with level of consciousness, lower blood pressure, and can depress the respiratory drive.

MOI. This is the mechanism of injury. We make a point to examine the car after a motor vehicle crash, and this can give important clues as to type of injuries there may be. If it was a fall, how far did they fall? If they were stabbed, how big was they knife?

MVC. This is a motor vehicle crash or collision. Years and years ago, it was known as a motor vehicle accident or MVA. The accident part was changed to crash or collision. To this day, people still refer to it as accident. When an intoxicated driver crashes his or her car, it is not an accident; it is a crash or collision.

myocardial infarction. This is medical terminology for heart attack. *Myo*=muscle, *cardial*=heart, and *infarction*=dying or death. Remember the mantra, "Time is muscle." This means no delays for getting a patient into the ED. The longer you delay, the greater and potentially more damage that occurs.

N

Narcan. This medication is a narcotic antagonist which means it reverses narcotic overdose or influence. One of the main reasons we use it is for heroin overdoses.

nare. This is one of your nasal openings. Both of them together are the nares.

nitroglycerin tablets/spray. This is medication used for chest pain suggestive of cardiac origin. The pain is caused by lack of oxygen to the cardiac tissues secondary to narrowing of the coronary arteries or blockage. Nitro is a vasodilator, meaning it will increase the size of the arteries and allow more blood flow and oxygen to the tissues. It can secondarily lower blood pressure, and we use it with great caution during a suspected myocardial infarction. There are two preparations we can use, spray form and small white tablet form. Both are administered beneath the tongue. A major contraindication is a person on erectile dysfunction drugs such as Viagra. They can have serious adverse reactions like major blood pressure drops.

normal saline. This is an IV solution infused into the vein through the IV catheter. It's used for fluid replacement which can temporarily raise blood pressure during blood loss. It doesn't have the oxygen carrying capability blood does; we also have to be very careful not to overload the system.

O

OD. This is the abbreviation for overdose.

oxygen tank. A small portable tank used to provide supplemental oxygen to a patient with difficulty breathing or in shock. Lack of oxygen can cause cardiac and brain cells to die. When we're in a patient's home, we need to ensure these small bottles are not left in a standing position. If the patient is lying on the floor and the bottle gets knocked over and hits them in the face, it's not going to be a good rest of the day for the patient or the crew.

P

periorbital ecchymosis. This is the bluish discoloration under both eyes, two black eyes. It's a sign that shows up with associated skull fracture and nasal fractures.

pinpoint pupils. This is the hallmark sign of narcotic influence. The pupils are extremely small. They resemble two periods in a sentence. This is something the patient has no control over. When someone has tiny pupils, and everyone else in the room has normal pupils, it's a billboard advertising what they've been doing. The droopy eyelids don't make their case any stronger.

pneumothorax. This is a collapsed lung. It can be spontaneous or from trauma. Trauma could include blunt, penetrating, or crushing. The primary sign is shortness of breath, and as it progressively gets worse, the skin color changes, becoming cyanotic or blue. Breathing is more labored and the person can die if it isn't treated. See tension pneumothorax.

postictal phase. This is the phase that follows a grand mal seizure. The patient may have mild disorientation to extreme combativeness. It can last from a couple minutes to several hours.

prone. This is a patient lying face down, on their stomach. It's a way we describe them positionally. The opposite is supine, face up.

pulmonary contusion. This is bruised lung tissue and collapse of the small air sacs in the lungs secondary to blunt force trauma to the chest. A major cause is motor vehicle crashes and collisions. Air exchange may be compromised leading to hypoxia. The patient will have trouble breathing and maybe cyanosis.

R

raccoon eyes. This is two black eyes. The patient resembles a raccoon face. It can be secondary to a skull fracture or broken nose.

radial pulse. Found on the thumb side of the wrist. If this pulse can be felt, the blood pressure is at least 80–90 for the top number. This means the patient is getting oxygenation to the brain and other vital organs. It's a great guide to quickly tell how bad your patient is when you first arrive. It's a true trick of the trade.

RGH. Regional General Hospital—This is a level one facility and capable of handling any type of emergency. There is no higher level of care facility.

rice krispies. This is air present in the subcutaneous layers of the skin. This is just below the level of the outer skin. In this case, it's referring to the skin over the chest. It can also be felt just under the skin in the neck or back. It has a characteristic of crackling feeling when palpated, thus the slang term of rice krispies. The actual term is subcutaneous emphysema. Subcutaneous referring to just under the skin and emphysema referring to trapped air.

ROSC. This is return of spontaneous circulation. It's the goal during cardiac arrest. It means a pulse has been restored.

RSI. Rapid sequence intubation—An elective procedure to put a patient to sleep and paralyze them in order to place an endotracheal tube into the trachea and take over the breathing process or protect the airway of severely injured person. RSI is only used for patients that have a respiratory drive. We generally have three reasons to consider this procedure: 1) Unable to maintain an open airway, maybe severe trauma; 2) unable to maintain a good oxygenation level, low SpO2 values, like maybe asthmatic or drowning; and 3) the anticipated clinical course of the patient, like a severely injured person that might go straight to surgery.

S

shock. This is inadequate perfusion to the tissues/cells resulting in vital organs shutting down or dying, heart, brain, and kidneys. The five types of shock include: 1) Hypovolemic—blood or fluid loss, 2) Cardiogenic—pump failure, 3) Anaphylactic—allergic reaction, 4) Septic—massive infection, and 5) Spinal—interruption of the spinal cord. People also confuse shock and anxiety. Anxiety is being upset after you wreck your car. At car crash scenes, someone might say, "That guy's in shock," and we notice he's smoking a cigarette and talking on a cell phone to his insurance agent. You don't die from having anxiety. You die from untreated shock.

slumper. This is a slang term used to describe a person pulled over on the side of the road and not moving. It's usually reported by a passing motorist who is concerned. Sometimes they will stop and most of the time they continue on. The person can be pulled over for any number of reasons, and occasional it's a genuine emergency.

SpO2 monitor. Measures the amount of oxygen saturation of hemoglobin. Hemoglobin is a protein molecule found in red blood cells and responsible for carrying oxygen molecules to the tissues. The SpO2 clip fits over the end of the finger and has an infrared light that measures the percentage of hemoglobin molecules saturated with oxygen molecules and displays the number in percentage values. We want the percentage to be over 94 percent. As a patient's saturation declines such as during the RSI procedure, we need to ventilate them in order to resaturate the hemoglobin molecules.

stent. This is a small mesh device placed in your blocked coronary artery and in the cath lab. It can allow for blood flow to be restored to the oxygen-deprived tissues and thus preventing permanent damage to the heart. The key is time. Our mantra in the prehospital arena when you're having chest pain is, "Time is muscle."

stridor. This is extreme narrowing of the airway in the back of the throat. It's a high-pitched sound similar to a deflating balloon as it's stretched restricting the air flow. It's a dangerous presentation and associated with inhalation burns and anaphylactic shock.

subcutaneous emphysema. This is rice krispies.

subdural hematoma. This is bleeding in the brain, a collection of blood beneath the dura level of the brain. It's a very small area right above the actual brain tissue. It qualifies as a (traumatic brain injury) TBI.

succinylcholine. This is medication used during the RSI procedure. It's a short-acting (up to eight minutes), muscle-paralyzing drug that renders the gag reflex ineffective. When the gag reflex is stimulated, it can raise the blood pressure precipitously causing significant injury to the brain. The medication is also known as sux.

sucking chest wound. This is an opening in the chest cavity usually from a penetrating source, stab wound, gunshot wound, or impalement. If the wound is larger than the tracheal opening, air will rush in during inhalation compromising the uninjured lung and interfering with the oxygenation process. The wound may have bubbling during the breathing phase. It is also known as an open pneumothorax.

supine. This is a person lying on their back, face up. It's a way we describe them positionally. The opposite is prone, face down.

sux. See succinylcholine.

T

tachypnea. This is medical terminology and means fast breathing. *Tachy*=fast, *pnea*=breathing.

TBI. Traumatic brain injury—This is a broad diagnosis of a probable brain injury that requires evaluation by CT scan.

tension pneumothorax. This is an immediate life-threatening condition that starts out as a simple pneumothorax which is collapsed lung. The normal breathing process has air going into the lung and back out through the mouth. When the lung is collapsed, the air goes in the chest, but now it cannot escape, it builds in the chest like a balloon until eventually the process stops and the patient dies. The lifesaving treatment is to insert the big needle and relieve the pressure. This is a temporary fix only. The patient will need a chest tube inserted once they get to the ED.

Time is Muscle. This is a saying we use to describe the priority for a patient having chest pain. We need to get them to the hospital ASAP in order for definitive treatment to be started. The quicker the treatment begins the less damage that can occur.

track marks. These are small needle marks from repeated injections along the vein tracks in the arms, hands, neck, and feet. This is evidence of IV drug use that includes heroin, methamphetamine, and cocaine. Sometimes the user will wear long sleeve clothing whenever in public to hide the marks.

truck bays. This is where we park the apparatus, the ambulance, the rescue, the fire engine.

12-lead EKG. A diagnostic assessment of the heart conducted when someone is having pain suggestive of cardiac origin. We place six electrodes on the chest, one on each arm and one on each leg which gives us a view of the entire heart and can see the heart attack happening in real time. Even though we only place ten electrodes on the patient, the LifePak 12 will add a virtual interpretation of two additional leads thus making it a 12-lead. We will call the hospital and declare a cardiac alert if we find obvious problems.

V

ventricular fibrillation. This is chaotic activity of the heart that does not produce a pulse, cardiac arrest. The patient requires CPR and defibrillation. The shock does not jump-start the heart as people think. It does the opposite of this. It stops all activity and hopefully allows the heart to restart on its own by its internal pacemaker.

Vicodin. This is a powerful narcotic pain reliever available by prescription only. It is taken orally, by mouth, and the user must be cautious with this drug as it can cause respiratory depression the same as heroin does.

V-fib. This is the shortened version of ventricular fibrillation.

vocal cords. This is the opening to the trachea and lungs. During the intubation process, as the laryngoscope is advanced down the throat, the first structure to be found is the epiglottis. Below this is the vocal cords and target for placing the endotracheal tube. The tube is inserted through this opening about 1–2 inches.

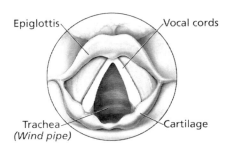

National Cancer Institute

W

watt seconds. This is one of two terms used to describe the energy delivered during ventricular fibrillation. One is watt seconds and the other is joules. They're both measurement of energies. We might start at 200 watt seconds and progress to a maximum of 360 watt seconds. We'll generally just call out a number when on scene and leave the watt seconds or joules part off.

X

x-ray. A radiologic assessment of bone and can be diagnostic for fractures.

Y

Z

zipper. This is a surgical scar through the center of the chest. It's indicative of cardiac bypass surgery. It's called a zipper because it sort of looks like a zipper.